KT-551-191

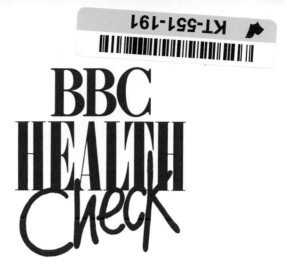

BBC HEALTH Check

WITH 14-DAY ACTION PLANS FOR BETTER HEALTH

DR BARRY LYNCH

BBC BOOKS

Published by BBC Books,
a division of BBC Enterprises Limited,
Woodlands, 80 Wood Lane, London W12 0TT
First published 1989

© Barry Lynch 1989

ISBN 0 563 21463 5

Set in 10/12½ pt Times by Ace Filmsetting Ltd, Frome
Printed and bound in Great Britain by Fletchers of Norwich
Cover printed by Fletchers of Norwich

CONTENTS

Acknowledgements	iv
Introduction: Choose Health!	1
1 You Are What You Eat	3
2 Losing Weight Healthily: the 14-Day Plan	17
3 Exercise: Start Moving	43
4 Is It Worth One More Puff? – Stop Smoking With the 14-Day Plan	58
5 Drinking Alcohol Sensibly	73
6 How to Avoid Heart Disease	89
7 Avoiding High Blood Pressure and Strokes	95
8 Coping With Stress	99
9 Women's Health	107
10 How to Cut the Risk of Cancer	121
11 Keeping Healthy As You Get Older	130
Useful Addresses	140
Further Reading	142
General Index	143
Index of Recipes	146
Healthcheck Diaries and Charts to Fill in	147–55

ACKNOWLEDGEMENTS

I should like to thank John Gurnett and Pam Cox of Radio 2 for organising the Radio 2 Healthcheck whence the idea of this book came. Thanks are also due to the presenters of Radio 2 who helped with the book: Gloria Hunniford, Jimmy Young, Derek Jameson, Adrian Love, John Dunn, David Jacobs and Ken Bruce.

I am very grateful to Dr Eleanor Carlson who devised the 14-day Diet Plan and to the Health Education Authority for their helpful comments on the whole manuscript. I would also like to thank Clive James, of the Health Promotion Authority for Wales, who gave useful suggestions on the exercise plan.

My thanks also go to Susan Martineau and Suzanne Webber of BBC Books for their work and enthusiasm, to Ellis Nadler who drew the cartoons, to Jo Dennis for the diagrams on p. 112 and pp. 114–16, and to Roland Unwin who designed the book.

I am indebted to Richard and Chrissie Trayler-Smith for their hospitality while I was writing this book and to Catrin Morgan who typed the manuscript in a breathtakingly short time.

INTRODUCTION: CHOOSE HEALTH!

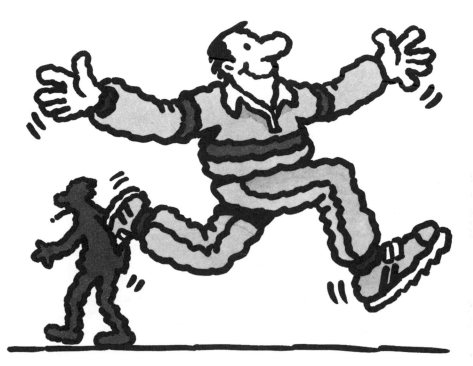

Are you healthy?

I don't mean 'have you just come out of hospital?' or 'do you have to take tablets?' or any question which means have you any illnesses. Being healthy doesn't just mean not being ill; it's a positive state, not just an absence of disease.

Do you feel tired all the time?
Do you feel you can't cope or do things get on top of you?
Do you feel at your peak?
Do you smoke?
Do you need to lose weight?
Do you think you drink too much?
Do you need to start taking exercise?

If the answer is yes to one or more of these questions, then this book can help you help yourself to better health. *Most people can do more for their own health than any tablet, doctor or hospital.*

If you follow the advice in this book:

- you'll greatly reduce the risk of a whole range of illnesses and life-shortening diseases.
- you'll be all you can be *now*. You'll be at the peak of your health. You'll feel tuned up and not sluggish; full of energy and not listless. You'll be at your most efficient at work, and you'll get the fullest enjoyment from your leisure.

The 14-day action plans in the book are your starter plans on the way to better health. With the 14-Day Weight-Loss Plan you'll rapidly feel the difference and, of course, in 14 days you can stop smoking and cut down drinking levels if you follow the guidelines in the appropriate plans. Remember, though, that these action plans are not just 14-day wonders but rather should help you get set on a plan for a long and healthy life. As you will see, the 14-Day Exercise Plan suggests fitness objectives for the weeks to follow and that should just be the beginning!

So many of the illnesses we suffer from and die from – before our time – are to a greater or lesser extent self-inflicted. By the lifestyle we lead we choose whether we greatly increase our chances of illness and premature death or whether we reduce our risk of those things to the absolute minimum.

Our health is truly in our own hands. We can gamble on our health in the future and mortgage it in the present. Or we can choose to be healthy now and have the best chance of keeping healthy. This book will help you with the choice. Choose health!

1 YOU ARE WHAT YOU EAT

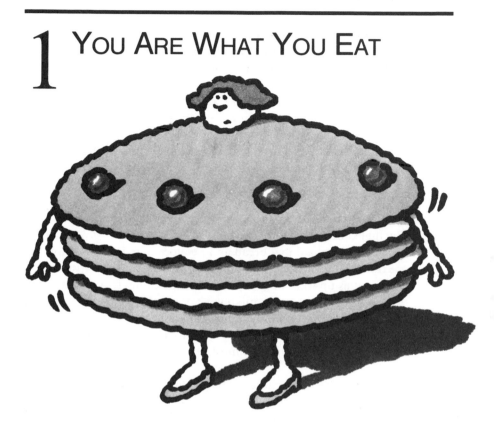

It's a very old adage but it's being proved more and more to be true by new scientific research that you really *are* what you eat.

Links between our health and our food have been known about for a long time – at least as far back as James Lind in the eighteenth century. He discovered that fresh oranges and lemons given to British sailors both treated and prevented scurvy.

It is, of course, common sense that what we put into our bodies through our mouths is going to have an effect on our health, but there's a confusing amount of information about the exact effects of different types of food.

WHAT IS KNOWN?

Sometimes, this mass of information we get about our food – from scientists, books and newspapers, radio and television and from the food industry itself – just serves to obscure one crucial fact. There is now overwhelming and worldwide, medical and scientific consensus on what constitutes a 'healthy' diet. And a 'healthy' diet is not only one which we can enjoy and will make us feel content, but also one which is associated with the longest and happiest life and with the lowest risks of a wide range of diseases. For it is now certain that many unpleasant and life-threatening diseases are associated with the pattern of eating that we follow in this country.

Is This Just Another Fad?

This is a very valid question, as advice about the food we eat has fluctuated in the last few decades.

It used to be said that bread and potatoes were fattening: now we're being encouraged to eat more of them because such starchy foods fill us up without giving us too many calories. We used to be exhorted to 'drinka pinta milka day': now we're being told to ensure that it's skimmed, or semi-skimmed at least. A good old fried British breakfast, it was claimed, would set you up for the day: now it's insisted that the thing it's most likely to set you up for is a heart attack.

Yes, the advice has changed. But no, it isn't a fad or fashion and you can be sure that the advice being given now is based on a huge amount of hard scientific evidence which is accumulating all the time.

It is this evidence which brought about the medical consensus on what constitutes a 'healthy' diet. Over the last decade or so, over 20 international reports on diet in the Western world have been in broad agreement. Enough is now known to recommend important changes in the way we eat. Those changes have been endorsed and encouraged by two British government reports in the last few years: NACNE (The National Advisory Council on Nutritional Education); and COMA (The Committee on the Medical Aspects of Food Policy).

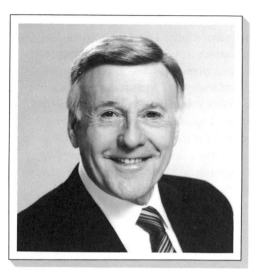

JIMMY YOUNG

I'm lucky – I happen to like food which is good for my health. I don't like fried food and I don't like sweet things. I don't eat much cheese and I practically never have any cream. My weight's been steady for many years. So I do eat food that seems to suit me and which is good for my health – but it's more by accident than design!

WHAT WILL WE GAIN IF WE DO CHANGE HOW WE EAT?

Many things! Among them will be a reduction in the risk of getting a range of diseases which our unhealthy diet either causes or makes us much more prone to. We can cut the risks of:

heart attacks
high blood pressure
strokes
several types of cancer
diabetes
gallstones
diverticular disease of the colon (a disease where small pouches, which can become inflamed, appear in the bowel wall)
constipation
being overweight

WHAT ARE THE CHANGES WE NEED TO MAKE?

The changes we need to make are encapsulated in four familiar little verses.

- Eat less fat.
- Eat less sugar.
- Eat less salt.
- Eat more fibre.

It's a pity the advice is summed up as three 'don'ts' and one 'do', but it is possible to follow the advice quite easily without ending up feeling that you're a medieval monk in Lent. Many people's traditional diet conforms to these principles. Good traditional Chinese food does and so does food of the Mediterranean basin: Southern French, Italian and Greek food. No one can say that healthy eating has to be boring. If we make some simple changes, good old British grub can be healthy too.

Now I said that the verses are quite familiar. What we need to know, though, is how to make practical sense of them. So here are some guidelines and suggestions for cutting down fat, sugar and salt and increasing fibre.

'EAT LESS FAT'

You may be saying, 'but I hardly eat any fat at all, I don't like it'. Well, it may come as a surprise but on average in this country we all get nearly 40 per cent of our food energy (calories) from fat – and that includes you! If you don't believe me, keep reading to see where the fat is found in our food and think of all the foods you ate yesterday which contained fat and yet perhaps didn't seem 'fatty'.

There are in fact two messages as far as fat and health are concerned: we need to eat less fat overall; and, in particular, we need to cut down on saturated fat. If we do that we can even increase a little the unsaturated fat we eat – always providing that we have reduced our fat consumption overall.

'Saturated' is a chemical term referring to the state of the hydrogen bonds which link the fat molecules together. 'Polyunsaturated' fat has a different chemical structure, with looser hydrogen bonds. (There's also 'monounsaturated' fat – olive oil is rich in this type of fat.) But you don't need to bother about chemistry; you just need to know where these different types of fat are found.

Saturated fats (or saturates) are:
- invariably solid at room temperature
- mostly found in fats of animal origin.

Butter, lard, the fat on steak and bacon, and double cream (remember the more solid or thicker cream is, the more fat there is in it) are examples of foods which are rich in saturated fat.

Polyunsaturated fats (or polyunsaturates) are:
- invariably liquid at room temperature
- mostly found in fats of plant origin.

Sunflower and most other oils, fatty fish like herring and mackerel, and most nuts are examples of foods which are rich in polyunsaturated fat.

(Butter does contain polyunsaturates and sunflower oil some saturates, but the main fat in each, by far, is the opposite.)

The problems of eating too much fat

Saturated fats in the diet increase the level of cholesterol in the bloodstream whereas polyunsaturated fats, in small doses, tend to decrease the level of cholesterol. Monounsaturated fats appear to have no effect on the level. If we have a high level of cholesterol in the blood, then our arteries are more liable to fur up, making strokes and heart attacks more likely. Too high a level of fat in the diet is also linked to various cancers of the intestine. And, of course, fat makes us fat – weight for weight it contains twice the calories of protein or carbohydrate – and being overweight contributes to a number of health problems too (see Chapter 2).

On average we eat four times as much saturated fat as polyunsaturated, so if we cut down on our fat intake across the board we will automatically take in less cholesterol-inducing saturated fat.

In the average British diet, here's where most of the fat comes from:
25 per cent from meat and meat products
21 per cent from butter and margarine
14 per cent from cooking oils and fats
11 per cent from milk
7 per cent from biscuits, cakes and pastries
7 per cent from cheese and cream
15 per cent from other foods.

The official government target is that we should, over the next decade, reduce our fat consumption by at least a quarter. This should not be so difficult to achieve as the guidelines below show.

Cutting down the fat from meat and meat products

■ Meat products like pies, pasties, sausages, pâtés and salami can be very high in fat. Half the calories in a sausage may be fat; nearly two-thirds of the calories in a meat pie may be fat. Choose lower-fat versions of these products which are now available everywhere or, better still, eat lean meat that you can identify as such.
■ Choose lean cuts of meat and trim off visible fat.
■ Choose white chicken or turkey meat and remove the skin.
■ Eat more white fish as it is low in fat. Fatty fish like herring and mackerel is low in saturated fat. Choose canned fish, like tuna and sardines, packed in brine rather than oil.
■ Always grill rather than fry – this reduces fat content greatly.
■ When cooking mince, choose the leanest you can buy.

Cutting down the fat from butter and margarine

■ Spread butter or margarine as thinly as possible.
■ Think of switching from butter to margarine labelled 'high in polyunsaturates' such as sunflower margarine. If you still use the same amount you won't have reduced your total fat intake, but you will have increased your polyunsaturated fat intake while reducing that of saturated fat. Margarine is, of course, easier to spread thinly.
■ Think of switching to low-fat spreads such as Gold or Outline. These contain only half the fat of any butter or margarine. I find the low-salt Gold very pleasant and buttery tasting. An interesting new product on the market is Shape Sunflower Spread – a low-fat spread which is also high in polyunsaturates.

Cutting down the fat from cooking oils and fats

■ Switch from hard cooking fats to oils. Again, this will decrease your saturated fat intake rather than your total intake as long as you switch to an oil which is high in polyunsaturates and low in saturates like Sunflower, Safflower or Groundnut.

- Avoid 'unnamed' oils labelled 'vegetable oil'. It is possible that these could contain the cheaper palm or coconut oils, which are unusually high in saturates for fat of vegetable origin.
- Olive oil is not only healthy (high in monounsaturates) but also strongly flavoured and can therefore make its mark in a dish in very small quantities.
- Grill rather than fry.
- If you do want to fry – an onion, for example – try 'dry-frying' in a heavy non-stick pan. You'll find that you can cook with no oil at all (add a little water if it starts to stick). Alternatively use the minimum amount of oil possible – you can fry an onion in one or two teaspoonfuls of oil.
- When you're making chips, you can cut down the fat they absorb by up to a half if you cut them thickly and fry them quickly in hot oil. Cutting the chips thickly means that weight for weight there's a lower surface area to absorb the fat. Frying them quickly cuts the fat content because hot oil doesn't seep into the chips as much as cooler oil. Don't keep re-using oil as heating it causes it to become more saturated. Always shake off as much oil as possible and, before serving, drain the chips on kitchen paper to get rid of any remaining fat.

Cutting down the fat from milk

It may be a surprise that milk is a significant contribution to the fat content of our diet. Ordinary silver-top (or full-cream) milk is 4 per cent fat and this is mostly saturated. This seems quite low but it's significant because we drink quite a lot of milk. If we drink, say, just less than one pint (600 ml) of full-cream milk a day – 6 pints (3.5 litres) a week – then we are consuming as much fat as there is in half a pint (300 ml) of double cream. Even half a pint (300 ml) of milk a day is the equivalent of drinking a pint (600 ml) of single cream a week.

- Skimmed milk contains virtually no fat at all but still has all the protein and calcium of ordinary milk. It is a little thin and so may take some getting used to. People who have got used to it often say they prefer its fresher, cleaner taste.

■ Semi-skimmed milk has only half the fat of ordinary milk and is a good compromise. You and your family can switch to this with no problem at all but one thing that should be mentioned is that children under two derive many of their calories from milk; it's wise to give them whole milk until this age and then get them used to semi-skimmed up to the age of five (providing the rest of their diet is adequate). After the age of five skimmed milk is fine. If you drink a lot of milk, your long-term aim should be to change eventually to skimmed milk.

Cutting down the fat from biscuits, cakes and pastries

Again, you may be surprised that these products contain fat in significant quantities. However, they do and this fat is usually high in saturates (even vegetable oils can be 'hydrogenated' to make them into hard fats for mixing with flour).

■ Try to cut down on these products which are basically just sweetened fat. Fresh fruit and dried fruits are healthier alternative snacks.

Cutting down on the fat from cream and cheese

■ Cream contains very significant quantities of fat, which is mostly saturated, and so should be reserved for occasional treats. Double cream, with 48 per cent fat, should definitely be a 'sometimes' food – just on your birthday perhaps! Whipping cream is 35 per cent fat and single cream is 18 per cent fat.
■ Try low-fat substitutes for cream such as low-fat natural yoghurt which is virtually fat-free. Make your own fruit yoghurt with this and fresh fruit.
■ Fromage frais or fromage blanc is made from skimmed milk and is creamy rather than cheesy as its French name suggests. It is delicious with fruit and makes very good fruit fools. It comes in tubs of 1 per cent and 8 per cent fat varieties. The latter has a little added cream for extra richness, but it's still less than half the fat of single cream and it's thick and spoonable. A spoonful or two of this higher-fat version is a perfect substitute for fresh cream in cooking.

(Note that if the writing on the tub is in French, it may talk about the 'fat content' or 'matière grasse' being perhaps 40 per cent. This is a different measure to the British 1 or 8 per cent as it refers to the percentage of fat of the contents *minus* the water it contains. The British measurement is consistent with all the other percentages in this book.)

- Greek-style yoghurt is delicious and tempting even to those who say they don't like low-fat natural yoghurt. It is, however, higher in fat content at 8–10 per cent fat. You can add it to hot dishes and, unlike low-fat natural yoghurt, it doesn't curdle if you add it gradually and stir well between each addition. If you want to cook with the latter, a teaspoonful of cornflour mixed with a little milk and stirred in will stabilise it.

- Cheese contains significant fat, which again is mostly saturated: Cheddar cheese is about 33 per cent fat; Stilton about 40 per cent fat; cream cheese about 50 per cent fat. Soft cheeses tend to contain less fat: Camembert, Brie and Edam are all about 23 per cent fat. These last three should be your choices if you want to reduce your fat intake from cheese. The reason for their lower fat content is that as soft cheeses they contain more water and so less fat, ounce for ounce.

- Cottage cheese is only about 4 per cent fat, so if you like it you're really on to a winner.

- Try the new half-fat Cheddar-type cheeses which are about 14 per cent fat. Some of them are rather bland but they seem to be improving all the time.

Cutting down the rest of the fat in your diet

- Nowadays, a significant contribution to the fat in our diet comes from salted snacks – crisps and all those strangely-shaped objects like tubes. The food industry tends to give us our fat as either sweetened fat or salted fat! Cut down on these snacks and go for the lower-fat versions which are now being produced.

- On the whole eggs are not a very significant contribution to the fat in our diet. It's true that egg yolks are high in cholesterol but it is the overall amount of saturated fat in our diet that pushes up the amount of cholesterol in our blood as our body uses saturated fat to manufacture cholesterol. The amount of cholesterol produced by egg yolks is fairly insignificant (provided you're not eating a dozen or more eggs a week, of course!). Three eggs a week is the recommended maximum number to aim for.

'EAT LESS SUGAR'

Can you believe that you eat a hundredweight of sugar a year or getting on for 2 lb (just under a kilo) a week? No? Well, that's what the average consumption is in this country. Each of us eats in a week what one person a hundred years ago ate in one year. Half of this sugar comes out of a packet and we add it ourselves to food. The other half comes ready-added to fizzy drinks and sweet confections, but it's also added to breakfast cereals, sauces, chutneys and tinned vegetables. If you start to read the ingredients' labels on food, you'll be surprised where sugar is added.

It's been suspected that the increased consumption of refined sugar is linked to various Western diseases such as heart disease. One professor of nutrition has labelled it pure, white and deadly. But direct links between sugar and those diseases have not been proved. What is certain, though, is that sugar is one of the reasons why so many of us – perhaps half of us – in this country are overweight. And it is being overweight, as we see in the next chapter, that increases the risk of a whole range of diseases.

In nature, sugar comes bound up with fibre – as in fresh fruit, for example. As fibre is bulky and filling, it's impossible to eat large quantities of sugar when it comes in this combination. In the manufacturing process, however, sugar is refined and concentrated and we can eat a large quantity of it before we feel full.

Sugar is often, aptly, described as containing 'empty calories'. It has no nutrients – just calories. It's a myth that you need sugar for energy because all food can be converted by your body into energy. Calories are a measure of that energy and most of us are only too well aware that all food contains calories!

It is also a myth that brown sugars are better for you than white; they're not – sugar is sugar. Molasses, glucose, dextrose, honey and syrup and treacle all amount to the same thing – sugar.

The ideal is to reduce your sugar consumption by half and here are some painless ideas to help you do it.

Ways you can begin to reduce your sugar intake

- Wean yourself off sugar in tea and coffee. Even if you have a sweet tooth, you can enjoy tea and coffee without sugar. I know because I now can't drink either with sugar yet, a few years ago, used to think I couldn't drink coffee without sugar and, a few years before that, couldn't drink tea without it either. This is a simple change to reduce your sugar consumption for life.
- Cut down on sweet snacks, biscuits and chocolate. Eat more fresh fruit instead.
- Choose tinned fruit packed in natural fruit juice rather than those in cloying sugar syrups.
- Reduce or completely cut out the sugar you add to your breakfast cereal. Check the ingredients of your family cereal. Many, including some of those promoted as 'healthy', have significant amounts of added sugar (and sometimes added salt as well). Choose one that doesn't have either.
- Read the labels on all manufactured food and if possible choose the ones which have reduced sugar content.
- Try cutting down the sugar in your favourite recipes: with most things, it's possible to reduce the sugar by up to a half with no less enjoyment.

'EAT LESS SALT'

We all eat far more salt than we need – perhaps as much as ten times more. On average, we each eat about ½ oz (12 g) a day – that's two whole teaspoonfuls! As with sugar, however, we don't completely control the amount of salt we eat. The biggest part of our salt intake is not what we add in cooking or at the table, but what is added by the manufacturer to processed food.

This abnormal level of salt intake is thought to be partly responsible for so many people in this country having high blood pressure (see Chapter 7). Some of us are sensitive to this unnecessary salt and it pushes up our blood pressure. The safest thing, therefore, is for us all to reduce our salt intake.

It would be almost impossible not to get enough salt. Even if we ate no salt and no processed food with salt, we'd still get about double our needs from the salt that occurs naturally in food.

We've trained ourselves (and our children) to like the taste of salt and to think that food doesn't taste of anything if we don't add it. But we can retrain our palates and it's surprising how quickly they can adapt. Once we begin to appreciate the natural tastes of food, then salted food begins to taste rather nasty.

Cutting down on the salt

- Read food labels. Again you'll be surprised where salt is added to food. Choose 'reduced salt', 'low salt' or 'no added salt' products when you can.
- Use less salt in your cooking. Herbs and spices, lemon juice and mustard can be used instead of salt to add flavour.
- Don't add salt to your food without tasting it first. You should aim eventually not to have a salt-cellar on your table.
- Cut down on crisps, salted nuts and other salted snacks.
- Cut down on food with a lot of added salt, like bacon.
- Salt is salt: sea salt crystals look nicer but they could still have the same effect on your body.
- Salt substitutes contain other chemicals like potassium chloride (salt is sodium chloride). They're expensive and it's much better to retrain your tastebuds.

'EAT MORE FIBRE'

Fibre is a carbohydrate found in all vegetable matter. It's what we used to call 'roughage'. Although we can't digest it, it's an important part of the food we eat because it helps the digestion process and keeps our bowels working normally. As we've been increasing the amount of processed foods we eat, the quantity of fibre in the national diet has gone down. This lack of fibre leaves us with room in our tummies for those fatty, sugary foods which make us fat.

The average British diet at the moment contains just over ⅔ oz (18 g) of fibre a day. This is very low compared with, for example, rural Africans whose daily intake is between 2–4½ oz (50–120 g) of fibre. During the Second World War, 1¼–1½ oz (32–40 g) of fibre a day was the average intake here. The consensus of medical opinion is that we should be eating at least 1¼ oz (32 g) of fibre a day – 50 per cent up on our present intake at least.

Many diseases which are common in the UK are associated with too little fibre in the diet. These include bowel cancer, constipation, diverticular disease (see p. 5), gallstones and diabetes.

Increasing the fibre in the diet tends to cause the level of cholesterol in the blood to fall and so reduce the risk of a heart attack. A high-fibre diet also enables us to reduce our fat and sugar consumption painlessly (see p. 17) and so reduce the chance of becoming overweight.

You may have heard of two drawbacks to a high-fibre diet, but these are easily overcome. It has been said that a large amount of fibre may interfere with the absorption of some essential minerals. People who have really gone over the top with the amount of fibre they eat have had some problems here. But you have to increase your fibre intake massively for this ever to be a problem – and increasing it by 50 per cent, or even doubling it, is not a worry. What's more, if you're eating a balanced diet you'll be getting enough of the minerals in question anyway – namely iron and calcium. You get iron from meat and vegetables, especially green leafy ones; and the vitamin C in fresh fruit and vegetables will help your body to absorb the iron it needs. You'd get more than enough calcium from half a pint of milk a day (full-fat, skimmed or semi-skimmed) and there's calcium in cheese, yoghurt and fromage frais and many other foods too.

Some fibre-rich foods, particularly pulses, peas and beans, can cause gas to be produced in the intestines giving the symptom of flatulence. As your body adjusts to more fibre, this problem should disappear. Throwing away the soaking water of dried peas and beans and cooking them in fresh water will help and the problem should be both minor and temporary. If it's really a nuisance for you, remember there are many other sources of fibre other than peas and beans.

Increasing your fibre

■ Eat more fibre-rich foods which include:

wholemeal bread
wholemeal flour
wholemeal pasta

brown rice
bulgar (or burghul) wheat
other grains (e.g. millet and buckwheat)
lentils
peas and beans (from baked to cannellini)
chick peas
sweetcorn
potatoes – baked in the jacket or boiled in the skin
green, leafy vegetables (e.g. spinach)
dried fruits (e.g. dried apricots).

- Try to start the day with muesli or a wholemeal breakfast cereal with no added sugar.
- Try to eat four slices of wholemeal bread a day (white bread contains some fibre, too, but only about a quarter of the quantity of wholemeal).
- Try to have a helping of one of the following with your main meal:

  potatoes (scrubbed not peeled) baked or boiled
  brown rice
  wholewheat pasta.

- Try to eat a portion of peas, beans or other pulses once a day.
- Eat at least one other portion of fresh vegetables a day.
- Eat two or three pieces of fresh fruit a day.

2 LOSING WEIGHT HEALTHILY: THE 14-DAY PLAN

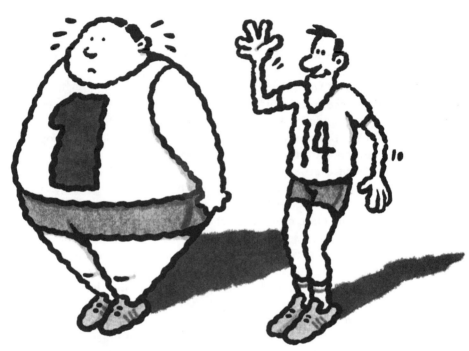

The easiest and surest way to lose weight is based on the same principles of eating healthily that we've just looked at.

Fat and sugar are the two culprits which make us overweight. They can both pack a lot of calories into a small space: they're calorie-packers. Fibre, on the other hand, is a great calorie saver as fibre-rich foods are filling but not fattening. They satisfy because they're bulky but they're not fattening because, weight for weight, they don't contain too many calories. So if you want to lose weight you need to:

- eat less fat
- eat less sugar
- eat more fibre.

No one is going to stick to a diet which gives them hunger pangs. And no one needs to! Later in this chapter is a 14-day weight-loss plan which is based on these principles and which is full of delicious enjoyable food. You'll see that losing weight need not be a penance. You can enjoy it!

ARE YOU OVERWEIGHT AND WHY SHOULD YOU WORRY?

Most people who are overweight know only too well they feel fat and that their body is trying to tell them something. Use the charts on page 19 to see whether or not you're overweight and, if so, how much over you are. If you *are* overweight, you're in good company. By the age of 25, 31 per cent of men and 27 per cent of women are substantially overweight and about half of middle-aged people in this country are above their ideal weight.

Being overweight is not just a matter of feeling uncomfortable. There are health risks too. Those who are overweight are more likely to have raised levels of cholesterol in their blood and are therefore more prone to heart attacks; they are more at risk of high blood pressure, diabetes and gallstone; they are more likely to suffer from various types of cancer and lung disease; and they may well get arthritis, bad backs and feel just generally tired and weary.

So, apart from all the other incentives you may have for wanting to lose weight – and they may be very important – one compelling reason is that you will improve your health and well-being and decrease the risks of suffering a wide range of illnesses.

THE KEY STEPS TO SUCCESSFUL WEIGHT-LOSS PREPARATION

Before you start on our 14-day weight-loss plan, it's a very worthwhile investment to spend a few days in preparation. This will greatly increase your chance of success, by developing your motivation, mobilising your will power and strengthening your resolve to keep off the weight you will lose.

Food diary

Keep a 'food diary' for a few days, including at least one weekday and one weekend day. This will give an accurate account of what you are actually eating at the moment – which will not, I promise

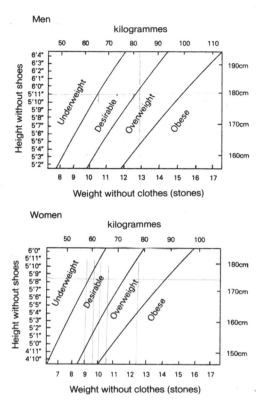

Find where you are on the chart by taking a line from the left-hand or right-hand side which gives your height. Follow this until it meets your weight line coming from the base or top of the chart. If you are perfect then the two lines meet in the middle of the 'acceptable' area. If you're not quite perfect then work out how far you are from the ideal.

you, correspond exactly with what you *think* you are eating. (An example of how a food diary might look is on pp. 20–1.)

Use your diary to identify your problem areas. Go through it and ask yourself about everything you've eaten: 'Does this contain fat?' 'Does it contain sugar?' 'What could I have eaten instead?'

Look particularly for when you were tempted to snack and work out some non-fattening snacks you could have instead – there are suggestions later in this chapter.

Watch out for the times you did something else at the same time as eating. If you were doing something like watching television while eating, remember you may be piling in food without even noticing it, let alone enjoying it.

FOOD DIARY

When	Where	What	With whom
7·45 am	Bedroom	2 digestive biscuits 1 tea with sugar	Alone
11·10 am	Office	1 doughnut 1 coffee with sugar	Catrin + Tessa
12·45pm	Canteen	2 sausages chips and peas, 1 tea with sugar	David + Tony
3·30pm	Office	Cream cake 1 tea with sugar	6 people
6·30pm	Home	Cheese and Onion Sandwich (white bread) 1 tea with sugar	Family
10pm	Home	Glass of lager - 1 pkt of crisps + 1 piece of pork pie	Husband

Why do you want to lose weight?

Think of your reasons for wanting to lose weight. Write them down. They will help your enthusiasm and determination. Try to think of at least ten; don't worry if some of them sound rather silly – they're your own, private reasons. For example:

I want to get into that pair of jeans again.
I want to get into that red dress again.
I want to appear on the beach next summer without blushing.

Activity	Hungry?	Mood	Comment
Getting dressed	Not really	Rush	Didn't think about it
Writing	Yes	Bored	Wish I'd waited till lunch
Talking	Yes	OK	More interested in the gossip than food
Talking John's Birthday	No	OK	Difficult to say no to the cream cake
Watching TV and talking	Yes	Tired	Eating without really noticing it
Watching TV	No	OK	Caught up in TV programme.

I want to learn to swim.
I don't want to be out of breath when playing with my grandchildren.
My husband/wife wants me to be slimmer.
I want to look good for my son's wedding next year.
My daughter is so slim and fit – I remember I was like that once and want to be like it again.

You get the idea!

Promise yourself

Make yourself a promise of how much weight you'll lose and think of giving yourself a reward for achieving it. It's best actually to write down your pledge. Make it a contract with yourself or with someone else, like your husband or wife or a friend. Rewards don't have to be extravagant to be effective. Simple rewards like a lie-in, breakfast in bed, someone else doing the washing-up, can all work well.

YOU'RE READY TO GO

You're now well-prepared to try our 14-day plan for a new you. Write down your present weight and in two weeks' time you'll have the pleasure of writing down your new weight and doing that pleasant subtraction to find out how much weight you've lost.

COPING WITH TEMPTATION

This diet plan is low in fat and sugar but high in fibre, so you shouldn't feel hungry – and tempted! Even when we're not hungry we may be tempted by a biscuit or a piece of chocolate, which in turn tempts us to another. If you know you have weaknesses in this direction, work out ways of coping with them. Here are some effective ones.

- Don't buy food which is fatty or sugary or is going to tempt you. Always write out a shopping list when you go to the supermarket and stick to it. Don't shop on an empty stomach.
- If you buy tempting food for other members of the family, lock it away or get them to hide it. Put it in a bag and write someone else's name on it.
- Have plenty of tempting non-fatty, non-sugary food around. Fresh fruit will be your best friend. Buy plenty of it. Carry an apple or another fruit around with you at all times. If you feel the need to have a chocolate, promise yourself that you'll eat an apple (or two!) first, then you'll be surprised at your strength to cope with temptation.
- Keep prepared sticks of carrot, cucumber, celery, pepper or radishes or florets of cauliflower in the fridge. Eat them when you feel like something savoury.

- Don't eat when you're doing something else like reading or watching television. Eat only at mealtimes if you possibly can. If you feel like snacking do something else instead – write a letter, call a friend, do some gardening or take a shower!
- At times of temptation look at your ten reasons for losing weight. Look at your contract and think of your reward.

Speeding up your Weight Loss

The very best way to speed up your weight loss is to combine the 14-day plan with some exercise – and keep exercising to help keep you slim (see Chapter 3). It not only helps burn up the calories but regular, sustained exercise also plays a part in increasing the 'tickover' speed of our bodies so that our metabolism is more efficient at keeping us slim. Regular exercise will also, of course, improve the fitness of our heart and the rest of our body.

Where Else can we Cut Calories?

In one word: alcohol. The average person will be taking perhaps 10 per cent of their daily calorie consumption from alcohol. This is drinking perhaps two or three drinks a day. You can cut these 200–300 calories at a stroke. You may decide you'd rather lose weight a little more slowly and continue to drink moderately (but see Chapter 5 for what 'moderate' means). It's important to remember that alcohol is 'empty' calories – supplying us with no nutrients. So don't substitute alcohol for food; if you want to try to lose weight on 1000 calories a day, you must add your calories from alcohol on top of this and accept that your weight loss will be slightly less rapid.

Very roughly – and as accurately as you need to know – one glass of wine and half a pint of beer and one single (pub measure) of spirits with a mixer are about 100 calories each. You should stick to only one measure of one of them a day if you want to lose weight. (Also, each of those measures contains one unit of alcohol.)

Getting to your Ideal Weight and Keeping There

- This 14-day plan is a healthy way of eating as well as an effective way of losing weight and you may repeat it as often as you wish. (Alternatively, there are five other two-week diet plans in the BBC book, *The BBC Diet*.)

- Start adapting your regular patterns of eating into more healthy and slimming ones by reading and putting into action the fat, sugar and fibre guidelines in the previous chapter. Incorporate as many as you can into your life and start to enjoy low-fat, lower-sugar, high-fibre food. That's the best way to guarantee that you won't put weight on again.

- Monitor your weight carefully. Weigh yourself once a week. Remember that fat creeps up slowly. If we put on only 4 oz (100 g) a week, that's nearly a stone (7 kg) in a year. If your weight does start creeping back on after the diet, observe the fat and sugar guidelines in the previous chapter more strictly.

- If you can't face life without any chocolate or fish and chips – don't despair! What you eat most of the time is what makes you thin or fat, healthy or unhealthy – not what you eat occasionally. Eat slim and healthy for 90 per cent of the time and you can gorge for the other 10 per cent. But remember which way round it is!

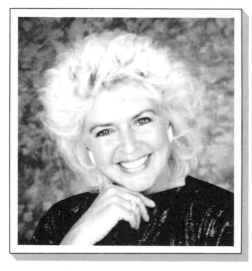

GLORIA HUNNIFORD

My Ulster childhood was full of delights like fried cabbage and bacon cooked in lard although we also ate good country bread and hearty soups and stews. Over the years I have made it a positive policy to cut out the fat in my diet and, even if I'm not rigidly good about it, I do make a conscious effort to watch what I eat.

THE BBC 14-DAY WEIGHT-LOSS PLAN DEVISED BY DR ELEANOR CARLSON

Our 14-day diet plan gives you 1250 calories a day – the ideal amount to help you lose those pounds yet keep your body well and nourished. However, if you are worried about any aspect of your health, check with your doctor before starting on this, or any other, diet.

As you will see, breakfast, a main meal and a snack has been worked out for each day to provide you with a delicious selection of menus. (You do not have to stick rigidly to each day's choice: if you wish you can 'mix and match' by choosing your three meals from the whole range of menus.) You are allowed unlimited cups of coffee or tea with skimmed milk but NO added sugar in beverages or on cereals and fruits. For your health's sake, try to cut down on the amount of salt you use in cooking (see p. 14).

Extra allowances included in the diet, but not described in the daily menus, are as follows:

- 3×5 fl oz (3×150 ml) glasses of dry white wine *per week*=300 calories
- 3 oz (75 g) polyunsaturated margarine *per week*=620 calories
- 2 oz (50 g) vegetable oil *per week*=500 calories or the equivalent in mayonnaise (see below)

The following are some approximate useful equivalents for the fat allowances to make sure you keep within the calorie limits allowed: 1×5 ml level teaspoon polyunsaturated margarine=1×5 ml level teaspoon vegetable oil=1×5 ml level teaspoon mayonnaise

Breakfasts for one person

As mentioned, unlimited cups of coffee or tea with skimmed milk are allowed with breakfast but NO sugar to be added to beverages or to cereals and fruits. Polyunsaturated margarine for spreading should come from the allowance outlined at the beginning.

Day 1	**Day 2**
½ grapefruit, unsweetened	5 fl oz (150 ml) unsweetened orange
2 Weetabix	*or* grapefruit juice
5 fl oz (150 ml) skimmed milk	1 Shredded Wheat
	5 fl oz (150 ml) skimmed milk

Day 3
2 oz (50 g) raspberries *or*
strawberries, unsweetened (if
tinned, in natural juice)
5 fl oz (150 ml) plain low-fat
yoghurt
1×1½ oz (40 g) wholemeal muffin

Day 4
1 pear
1 oz (25 g) branflakes
5 fl oz (150 ml) skimmed milk

Day 5
5 fl oz (150 ml) unsweetened orange
or grapefruit juice
2 slices wholemeal bread

Day 6
5 fl oz (150 ml) tomato *or* V8 juice
(available in healthfood shops)
1 poached *or* boiled egg
1 slice wholemeal bread

Day 7
½ grapefruit, unsweetened
4 oz (100 g) mushrooms, cooked in
a non-stick pan with no added fat
1 slice wholemeal toast

Day 8
5 fl oz (150 ml) unsweetened orange
or grapefruit juice
5 oz (150 g) porridge (2 oz (50 g)
oats and 3 fl oz (100 ml) water)
5 fl oz (150 ml) skimmed milk

Day 9
1 whole small *or* ½ large banana *or*
1 peach
1 wholemeal muffin

Day 10
1 apple, grated
1 Weetabix
5 fl oz (150 ml) skimmed milk

Day 11
½ grapefruit, unsweetened
1 oz (25 g) unsweetened muesli
5 fl oz (150 ml) skimmed milk

Day 12
½ banana, sliced
1 Shredded Wheat
5 fl oz (150 ml) skimmed milk

Day 13
1 orange *or* tangerine
1 boiled egg
1 grilled tomato
1 slice wholemeal toast

Day 14
5 fl oz (150 ml) tomato juice
4 oz (100 g) mushrooms, sliced and
'simmered' without fat in a non-
stick pan
1 slice wholemeal toast

Snack meals and main meals for one person

Again, don't forget to take your polyunsaturated margarine for spreading from your allowance.

Day 1
2 slices wholemeal French almond toast (see p. 29)
1 piece of fresh fruit

stir-fried beef with vegetables (see p. 30)
1 oz (25 g) brown rice (uncooked weight)
3 oz (75 g) green beans (if tinned, in unsalted water)
1 baked banana (see p. 41)

Day 2
2 slices wholemeal bread
1 oz (25 g) lean ham
lettuce and tomato
grapes (as many as you like)

5 oz (150 g) lean pork chop
5 oz (150 g) boiled new potatoes
3 oz (75 g) leeks
2×15 ml tablespoons Hollandaise sauce (see p. 40)

Day 3
7 oz (200 g) tinned tomato soup
orange and onion ring salad (see p. 39)
1 wholemeal roll

chicken pasta salad (see p. 37)
3 oz (75 g) ice-cream

Day 4
mixed salad (see p. 37)
1 wholemeal roll
mayonnaise and spread from allowance
1 small low-fat yoghurt

chilli con carne y frijoles (see p. 31)
tomato and lettuce salad
2 crispbreads
apricot fool (see p. 42)

Day 5
2 slices wholemeal bread
2 oz (50 g) white turkey meat
lettuce and tomato

pasticcio (see p. 32)
mixed salad (see p. 37)

Day 6
2 oz (50 g) hummus
1 wholemeal pitta bread
1 tomato
1 apple

2 savoury filled pancakes (see p. 33)
3 oz (75 g) spinach (fresh or frozen)
4 oz (100 g) mixed fruit salad (see p. 41)

Day 7
2 slices wholemeal bread
1½ oz (40 g) Cheddar cheese
1 pear

5 oz (150 g) lean rump steak, grilled
6 oz (175 g) jacket potato
green bean salad (see p. 38)

Day 8
walnut and apple salad (see p. 38)
4 oz (100 g) cottage cheese
2 crispbreads

6 oz (175 g) steamed white fish
2×15 ml tablespoons Hollandaise
   sauce (see p. 40)
6 oz (175 g) new potatoes
devilled carrots (see p. 34)

Day 9
6 oz (175 g) jacket potato
4 oz (100 g) baked beans in tomato
   sauce
1 small low-fat fruit yoghurt

salad supreme (see p. 38)
4 oz (100 g) liver, grilled *or* cooked
   in a non-stick pan with no added
   fat
3 oz (75 g) Brussels sprouts

Day 10
2 slices wholemeal bread
egg salad (1 hard boiled egg plus
   mayonnaise from allowance)
fresh fruit: apricot, peach, plum

spicy rice with cashew nuts (see p. 36)
carrot salad with mustard seeds (see
   p. 39)

Day 11
7 oz (200 g) hearty lentil soup (see
   p. 29)
2 crispbreads
1 oz (25 g) Camembert-type cheese

¼ chicken, skinned and grilled
6 oz (175 g) new potatoes
peas and water chestnuts (see p. 35)

Day 12
2 slices wholemeal bread
tuna salad (see p. 39)
1 pear

prawn and okra gumbo (see p. 34)
2 oz (50 g) brown rice (uncooked
   weight)
3 oz (75 g) cauliflower

Day 13
6 oz (175 g) cheese and tomato
   pizza
fresh fruit

tagliatelle al limone (see p. 35)
3 oz (75 g) broccoli

Day 14
'a taste of Araby' (see p. 40) with
   hard boiled egg wedges

5 oz (150 g) lean lamb chop
yoghurt with walnuts and fresh
   coriander (see p. 41)
6 oz (175 g) new potatoes
garlicky courgette (see p. 36)

French almond toast (Serves 1)

1 egg, beaten
8 fl oz (250 ml) semi-skimmed milk
2 thick slices wholemeal bread
1×15 ml tablespoon almonds, finely chopped
pinch of nutmeg

Blend the milk into the beaten egg. Pour this mixture over the bread and allow to stand until all the moisture has been absorbed.
　Heat a non-stick pan and brush lightly with polyunsaturated oil. On a medium heat brown the bread on one side and then turn. Sprinkle with the nutmeg and chopped almonds. Cook until both sides are brown and the slice has become firm. Test by inserting a knife into the centre of the slice. If it comes out clean it is cooked. Do not overcook or it will become dry.

Hearty lentil soup (Serves 4)

9 oz (250 g) dried brown lentils (the flat, greeny brown ones)
1½ pints (900 ml) cold water
2 bay leaves
3 oz (75 g) onion, chopped
2 cloves garlic, peeled and crushed
4×5 ml teaspoons olive oil
1×15 ml tablespoon tomato purée *or* 1 fl oz (25 ml) sieved tomatoes
salt and pepper
2–3×5 ml teaspoons vinegar
parsley for garnish

Wash and soak the lentils in warm water for about 1 hour. Drain. Add the cold water and the bay leaves and bring to a boil. Skim.
　Sauté the onions and garlic in the olive oil and add to the lentils. Simmer for 30–45 minutes until the lentils are soft.
　Add the tomato, salt, pepper and vinegar and simmer for 10 more minutes until the flavours blend. Sprinkle with chopped parsley before serving.

Stir-fried beef with vegetables   (Serves 4)

Although this simple recipe uses beef, it is also possible to make it with lean pork or liver and the vegetables may be varied according to seasonal availability.

1 lb (450 g) skirt steak
1 oz cube (25 g) ginger root, shredded
2 cloves garlic, peeled and crushed
1×5 ml teaspoon lemon juice
2×15 ml tablespoons soy sauce
1×15 ml tablespoon polyunsaturated vegetable oil
½ medium green pepper, cut in strips
3 oz (75 g) broccoli, cauliflower, carrots *or* green beans
1 medium onion, cut into thin wedges
2 medium tomatoes, cut into wedges
2 spring onions, bulb and green chopped into 1 in (2.5 cm) lengths

Remove the fat and membrane from the beef and cut across the grain into thin slices 2 in (5 cm) long. Place in a shallow dish. Mix the ginger, garlic, lemon juice and soy sauce and pour over the meat. Stir until each slice is coated with the mixture.

Heat half the oil in a wok or deep-sided frying-pan and stir-fry the meat slices over high heat for 2 minutes or until the colour changes. Remove the meat with a perforated spoon and put on one side.

Add the remaining oil and all the vegetables, except the spring onions and tomatoes, to the frying-pan and stir-fry for about 1 minute. Then add the meat and any juices which have collected to the pan. Add the tomatoes and spring onion. Blend everything well.

Serve with brown rice.

Chilli con carne y frijoles   (Serves 4–6)
(Mexican chilli with meat and beans)

1 lb (450 g) dried red kidney beans
1 lb (450 g) lean beef, cut into cubes
1 pint (600 ml) beef stock
1 large onion, finely chopped
3–4×5 ml teaspoons medium chilli powder *or* a combination of chilli and
  paprika (vary amount according to taste)
¼×5 ml teaspoon crushed cumin seeds
salt to taste

Soak the beans overnight. Pour off the water and replace with about 2 pints (1.2 l) boiling water. Boil vigorously for 15 minutes. (This will destroy any toxins on the outside of the beans.) Turn down the heat and cook for 30 minutes. Drain.

In another pan, cover the beef with boiling beef stock and simmer for 1 hour. Then mix the chopped onion and half the chilli powder with the cumin and add to the beef.

Combine the beef and beans and simmer until the beef is tender. The beans should be soft but remain whole.

Add salt to taste and check the seasoning. Add the remaining chilli powder or a combination of chilli and paprika, depending on your preference for spicy, hot food.

Garnish with raw chopped onion before serving if wished.

Pasticcio   (Serves 3–4)
(baked macaroni with minced meat)

8 oz (225 g) lean minced beef
1 medium onion, finely chopped
1×14 oz (400 g) tin chopped
  tomatoes *or* 400 ml strained
  tomatoes
2 bay leaves
nutmeg and ground cinnamon to
  taste
salt and pepper
8 oz (225 g) wholewheat pasta quills

White sauce:
10 fl oz (300 ml) skimmed milk
1 egg, beaten
1 oz (25 g) plain flour
1 oz (25 g) polyunsaturated
  margarine
1 oz (25 g) Parmesan cheese, grated

Heat the milk gently without boiling. Melt margarine slowly in a
heavy-bottomed pan. Remove from heat and stir in flour
thoroughly. Then add ⅓ of the heated milk. Stir and add remaining
milk. Return to medium heat and stir until mixture begins to froth.
Remove from heat and stir in the beaten egg and a grating of
nutmeg. In a non-stick pan heat a drop of oil and cook the onions
until soft. Remove from the pan and keep in a warm place.
    Put the meat in the non-stick pan and cook over a medium heat
for about 20 minutes, stirring frequently. Remove from heat and
skim or drain off the excess fat. Add the onion, a grating of nutmeg
and ¼×5 ml teaspoon cinnamon and mix well. Cook until slightly
brown. Add the tomatoes and bay leaves and cook over low heat
for a further 15 minutes. Remove from heat and mix in 2 good
15 ml tablespoons of white sauce. Season.
    Meanwhile cook the pasta, according to the instructions on the
packet, until soft but firm. Drain. Add 2 good 15 ml tablespoons of
the white sauce and mix well.
    Put a layer of half the macaroni in a fire-proof dish. Pour half
the meat sauce over this followed by another layer of macaroni on
top. Cover with another layer of the meat, and pour the white sauce
over the top making sure it runs down around the edges of the dish.
Sprinkle the Parmesan cheese over the top and bake for about 40
minutes at gas mark 5, 375°F (190°C) when the top should be a
golden brown.
    Allow to set for a while before cutting into squares to serve.

Savoury filled pancakes   (Makes 8 pancakes)

For whichever filling you choose just combine the ingredients and
gently heat the mixture. You can either use both fillings or, if
preferred, pick one and make double the quantity.

Pancake batter:
5 oz (150 g) wholemeal flour *or* half wholemeal and half plain white flour
1 egg, beaten
10 fl oz (300 ml) skimmed milk
1×15 ml tablespoon vegetable oil

Fillings:

6 oz (175 g) white fish (cod, haddock, halibut), steamed, skinned and flaked	*or* 4 oz (100 g) left-over roast chicken, diced
10 fl oz (300 ml) white sauce made with skimmed milk (see p. 32)	4 oz (100 g) tinned sweetcorn
1×5 ml teaspoon curry powder	10 fl oz (300 ml) white sauce made with skimmed milk (see p. 32)
salt and pepper	salt and pepper

Mix the flour, egg and milk to a smooth batter. Allow to stand for
about 30 minutes. Stir well before using.

Heat a teaspoon of oil in a non-stick frying-pan. Pour in a little
of the batter. Tip the pan so that the batter is evenly distributed.
Turn over when air holes appear, and the surface is set. Brown on
the other side. Turn on to greaseproof paper and keep warm.
Continue until you have 8 pancakes, using a tiny amount of oil in
the pan each time.

Evenly distribute the hot filling between the pancakes, roll and
garnish with chopped parsley.

Prawn and okra gumbo   (Serves 4)

1×15 ml tablespoon olive oil
1 large onion, finely chopped
1 clove garlic, peeled and crushed
1 medium green pepper, de-seeded and chopped
1×14 oz (400 g) tin chopped tomatoes
1 bay leaf
½×5 ml teaspoon dried thyme
2 whole cloves
8 oz (225 g) okra cut into ½ inch (1 cm) long rounds
1 lb (450 g) cooked, peeled prawns
1×15 ml tablespoon chopped parsley for garnish
cayenne pepper (optional)

Heat the olive oil in a non-stick pan and add the onion, garlic and green pepper. Cook gently until soft. Add the tomatoes, bay leaf, thyme and cloves and bring to a boil. Turn the heat down and simmer for 15 minutes.

Add the okra and cook for 5 minutes. Add the cooked prawns and cook for another 5–10 minutes. The okra and prawns should both keep their colour.

Devilled carrots   (Serves 2)

2–3 medium carrots
1×5 ml teaspoon vegetable oil
½×5 ml teaspoon paprika
2×5 ml teaspoons lemon juice *or* vinegar

Cut the carrots into julienne strips and in a little water steam in a non-stick pan until just tender. Heat the vegetable oil, add the paprika and fry for several minutes, just long enough to bring out the flavour. Add the carrots and lemon juice and stir until well coated. Serve hot.

Tagliatelle al limone (noodles with lemon sauce)   (Serves 1)

> 2–3 oz (50–75 g) dried tagliatelle *or* spaghetti (fresh is better and quicker to
>   cook but more expensive)
> zest and juice of ½ lemon
> ½–1 clove garlic, finely chopped (optional)
> 2×15 ml tablespoons Greek-style yoghurt (sheep *or* cow's)
> ¼ oz (10 g) freshly-grated Parmesan cheese
> black pepper

Cook the pasta as directed on the packet. Peel the zest of the lemon finely, leaving behind the white pith. Chop finely. Squeeze the lemon. Add the lemon juice, zest and garlic to the yoghurt and heat gently. (Unlike normal low-fat yoghurt, Greek-style yoghurt does not separate when heated gently but do *not* boil.)

When the pasta is cooked, drain well and add to the lemon sauce. Mix well. Serve on a heated plate and sprinkle with the Parmesan and pepper.

Peas and water chestnuts   (Serves 1)

Water chestnuts are not really nuts but tubers (just as potatoes are). Four chestnuts weigh about 1 oz (25 g) and contain about 14 calories. Water chestnuts can be added to other vegetables and salads to give texture and variety.

> 3 oz (75 g) peas, fresh or frozen
> 4 tinned water chestnuts
> mint to garnish

Drain tinned water chestnuts and slice. Add the chestnuts to the peas and cook in very lightly salted or unsalted water.

Spicy rice with cashew nuts   (Serves 4)

> 1×15 ml tablespoon vegetable oil
> 1 medium onion, finely chopped
> 3 whole cardamoms
> 7 oz (200 g) brown rice
> 2 whole cloves
> 1 inch (2.5 cm) stick of cinnamon
> 1×5 ml teaspoon curry powder
> 15 fl oz (450 ml) water
> 3 oz (75 g) cashew nuts (unsalted)
> 2 medium tomatoes, chopped

Heat half the oil in a non-stick saucepan which has a tight-fitting lid. Add the onion and fry until golden brown. Remove the outer husks of the cardamoms and keep the seeds. Discard the husks. (For a milder flavour you can use whole cardamoms but remove them before serving.) Add the rice and the spices and stir until the rice is a good fawn colour.

Boil the water and add to the rice along with a little salt, stir, cover and cook for about 30 minutes or until all the water has been absorbed.

In a heavy-bottomed pan heat the remainder of the oil. Fry the cashew nuts on medium heat until they begin to colour. Add the cashew nuts and chopped tomatoes to the cooked rice and stir. Replace the lid and allow to sit and gently heat for a few minutes so that the tomatoes get properly hot and the flavours blend.

Remove the whole spices and fork the rice into a dish to serve.

Garlicky courgette   (Serves 1)

> 1 large courgette
> 1 small clove garlic, peeled and crushed

Place a drop of oil (from the allowance) in a non-stick pan. Add the garlic and fry until brown. Coarsely grate the courgette and add to the pan. Stir frequently. Cook for 2 minutes or until the courgette is heated through. Do not overcook or the courgette becomes limp and watery. Season to taste.

Chicken pasta salad   (Serves 1)

2 oz (50 g) wholewheat pasta twists
5 oz (150 g) chicken breast
2 fl oz (50 ml) dry white wine *or* water
2 oz (50 g) broccoli spears
2 oz (50 g) raw mushrooms, sliced
1 oz (25 g) red pepper, de-seeded and coarsely chopped
1 spring onion, chopped
juice of ½ lemon
a pinch of marjoram, fresh *or* dried
salt and pepper to taste

Cook the pasta in unsalted or very lightly salted water until soft but firm. Drain and toss in 2×5 ml teaspoons olive oil from allowance.

Skin and poach the chicken breast, for 30 minutes, in the wine in a tightly covered container in the oven at gas mark 4–5, 350°–375°F (180°–190°C). Cool. Remove any bones and cut into bite-sized chunks. (Alternatively, left-over roast chicken can be used.)

Cook the broccoli just long enough for it to become tender but still retain some crunch. Rinse in cold water and drain. Leave to cool.

Put the pasta, chicken and all the vegetables in a large bowl. Add marjoram, salt and pepper to taste. Add lemon juice and toss.

Mixed salad

Any combination of the following ingredients may be used:

Chinese cabbage, lettuce, radicchio, mushrooms, green and red pepper, onion, tomato.

Wash and prepare all the salad vegetables and toss with some lemon juice to taste. Alternatively mix in some of the mayonnaise from your allowance. You can eat as much of these salad ingredients as you like without affecting the rules of the diet.

Green bean salad   (Serves 2–3)

> 8 oz (225 g) whole green beans, fresh *or* frozen
> ½ medium green pepper
> ½ medium red pepper
> 2 slices red onion
> 2 oz (50 g) raw mushrooms, sliced
> ¼ bunch watercress
> juice of ½ lemon
> 2×5 ml teaspoons olive oil

Cook the beans until 'al dente' (with a bit of bite left). Rinse in cold water and drain. Separate the onion rings and combine all the vegetables.

Mix the lemon juice and olive oil and pour over the vegetables. Toss until they are all coated.

Walnut and apple salad   (Serves 1)

> 1 apple, coarsely chopped
> 1 stick celery, chopped
> 1×15 ml tablespoon raisins
> 1 oz (25 g) walnuts, chopped
> juice of ½ lemon

Mix well and serve on a bed of salad greens.

Salad supreme   (Serves 1)

> 1 large carrot, grated
> ½ banana, sliced
> 1 oz (25 g) roasted peanuts (unsalted)
> lemon juice to taste

Toss all the ingredients together to mix and then serve.

Orange and onion ring salad   (Serves 1)

1 orange
2 slices of raw onion
lemon juice
salad greens (as much as you like)

Peel the orange and remove as much of the white pith as possible. Slice into rounds. Separate the onion rings. Pile everything on top of the salad greens and sprinkle with lemon juice.

Carrot salad with mustard seeds   (Serves 2)

2–3 carrots, finely grated
1×5 ml teaspoon olive oil
1×5 ml teaspoon dark mustard seeds
2×5 ml teaspoons lemon juice

Heat the olive oil and mustard seeds in a deep-sided pan until the seeds begin to pop. Allow to partially cool before pouring over the grated carrots.
   Add the lemon juice and mix well.

Tuna salad   (Serves 1)

½×7 oz (200 g) tin tuna, in brine
1 stick celery
1×5 ml teaspoon mayonnaise (from allowance)
cucumber slices to garnish

Drain and flake the tuna. Wash and then finely chop the celery. Mix tuna, celery and mayonnaise together and garnish with the cucumber slices.

'A taste of Araby' bulgar wheat salad   (Serves 4)

4 oz (100 g) cracked (bulgar) wheat
2 oz (50 g) spring onions, chopped
2 oz (50 g) parsley, chopped
½ oz (15 g) fresh mint, finely chopped
4 oz (100 g) tomatoes, chopped into cubes
1 fl oz (25 ml) olive oil
1 fl oz (25 ml) lemon juice
salt and pepper to taste

The bulgar wheat has already been cooked so all you need to do is reconstitute it by soaking in cold water for about 1 hour until swollen. Drain and squeeze out any excess moisture.

Put the wheat in a bowl and add the other ingredients. Stir and season to taste. Add more lemon juice for a very tart flavour.

Hollandaise sauce   (Serves 8)

5 fl oz (150 ml) mayonnaise
3 fl oz (85 ml) skimmed milk
2×5 ml teaspoons lemon juice

Stir the milk and mayonnaise together and heat gently in a non-stick pan. (Do not allow the mixture to boil.) Heat it for about 10 minutes, then remove from the heat, add the lemon juice and stir until well blended. Serve hot or cold.

This sauce can be used with vegetables or fish dishes. It is best to make the sauce fresh each time rather than keep it.

Yoghurt with walnuts and fresh coriander   (Serves 4)

10 fl oz (300 ml) low-fat plain yoghurt
1×15 ml tablespoon fresh coriander, finely chopped
1 spring onion, finely chopped
1 oz (25 g) shelled walnuts, roughly chopped
salt and pepper to taste

Put the yoghurt into a bowl and lightly whisk until creamy and smooth. Add the other ingredients and stir to mix. Allow to sit for 20 minutes before serving for the flavours to blend.

Baked banana   (Serves 1)

1 banana
1×5 ml teaspoon dark brown sugar
zest and juice of 1 orange
1×5 ml teaspoon desiccated coconut

Lightly brush a baking dish with polyunsaturated oil.
    Peel and slice the banana lengthwise and place in baking dish. Sprinkle with brown sugar. Add the zest and juice of the orange and the coconut.
    Bake in a moderate oven (gas mark 3, 325°F, 160°C) for 20 minutes.

Fruit salad   (Serves 1)

Any combination of the following ingredients may be used:

1 apple
1 orange
grapes
pear, peach *or* apricot
1 banana
unsweetened orange juice to mix

Clean and prepare your chosen fruit and moisten it with the orange juice. Toss it to mix and chill until needed.

Apricot fool   (Serves 4–6)

> 4 oz (100 g) dried apricots
> 8 fl oz (225 ml) low-fat fromage frais
> 5 fl oz (150 ml) low-fat natural yoghurt

Put the apricots in a small saucepan and cover with water. Bring to the boil slowly and then simmer gently for 10–15 minutes. Leave to cool. The apricots should absorb most of the juice.

Finely chop the apricots and their liquid in a liquidiser or food processor. Add the fromage frais and mix. Turn into a bowl and stir in the low-fat yoghurt until thoroughly blended. Serve in small bowls or glasses topped with a teaspoon of natural yoghurt.
Note Alternatives are: *Pineapple fool* made with 6–8 oz (175–225 g) fresh pineapple instead of the apricots; or *Passion fruit fool* made with the juice and pulp of 4 passion fruits and 4×5 ml teaspoons of caster sugar instead of the apricots.

3 EXERCISE: START MOVING

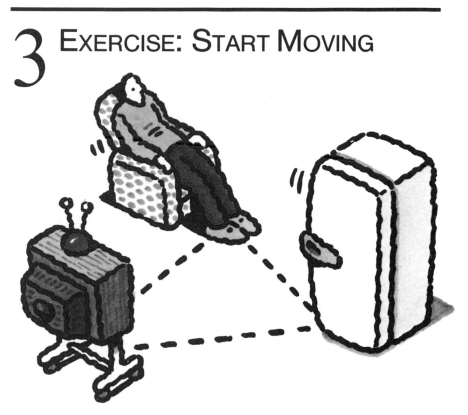

How much did your body move yesterday? I'm not talking about formal exercise, just everyday moving around. In an average day some of us do little more than walking a few yards from the front door to the car and perhaps another few yards up and down a corridor. The most energetic thing we may do in a day is brushing our teeth! Am I exaggerating? Well, perhaps a little – but not much. It's a very salutary lesson to keep a simple exercise diary for a day or two and see just how little movement we can get away with in the course of an average day. Try it and I'm sure you'll be surprised at the result. There's an example of how one might look on p. 44.

OUR FEET WERE MADE FOR WALKING ...

... and our bodies were made for exercising regularly. Our cavepeople ancestors had to exercise because they had to run and climb in order to get their food. Although we live in a push-button world

Exercise Diary

Time	Where was I?	What did I do?
7.00 – 7.30 7.30 – 8.00 8.00 – 8.30	In bed In bathroom In bedroom	Switched alarm off Showered, brushed teeth Dressed; turned over pages of the newspaper
8.30 – 9.00	In kitchen	Ate breakfast
9.00 – 9.30	In car	Walked 3 yards to car and 10 yards car to office
9.30 – 10.00	In office sitting at desk	Telephoned, wrote, walked 20 yds to loo
12.30 – 1.00	Eating sandwiches	Moving hands to mouth!
2.00 – 2.30	In office sitting at desk	Telephoning, writing walked 5 yds to another office twice.
5.30 – 6.00	In car	Walked 10 yds from office to car; 3yds from car to front door
6.00 – 6.30	In garden	Sitting
7.00 – 7.30	In kitchen	Eating and drinking - moving hands to mouth
8.00 – 8.30	In the sitting room	Watching TV pressing remote control switch!
10.00 – 10.30	In bed	Reading - turning pages
11.00 – 7.00	In bed	Asleep - tossing + turning

where we don't need to get out of our armchair even to change channels on the television set, our bodies are not adapted for it. We still have the same bodies which were designed for vigorous activity and our muscles and joints especially miss it when we don't exercise. Without exercise we're like badly-tuned engines which don't work efficiently, either physically or mentally.

EXERCISE IS FOR EVERYONE

'I'm no Daley Thompson,' you may be saying to yourself but exercise is normal and natural for us all – we're not talking about scaling Olympian heights. We all have what's called a 'fitness gap' – the difference between our present state of fitness and what it could be if we did what is really a normal amount of exercise. For most people, the gap is very wide so we're not talking about superhuman efforts – even regular walking will close that fitness gap significantly. (For someone like Daley Thompson, the difference between his potential fitness and his actual fitness is very tiny – the gap is very narrow.)

And remember we're not competing with anyone else – it's a matter of having the health and fitness which really should be ours by right.

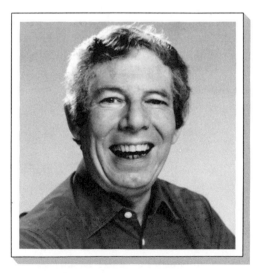

DEREK JAMESON
I'm a great believer in drinking lots of water and going easy on the booze. Most of my life I've been fighting a losing battle with the demon nicotine. Maybe I'll have more luck with exercise – it's certainly worth a bash, isn't it?

THE BENEFITS OF EXERCISE

Regular exercise really will bring you so many benefits.

- It will set you up for the day; you'll feel better, work better and have more energy.
- It will help you to sleep better and more soundly.
- It's a very good way of relieving stress; those giving up smoking will find it particularly helpful.
- It will help to keep your joints and muscles in good working order right into old age.
- It will strengthen your bones, so that there's less risk of osteoporosis, or thinning of the bones, as you grow older.
- It will improve your circulation so that more oxygen will reach all parts of your body.
- It will help you to lose weight, and achieve or maintain your ideal weight.
- It will cause the percentage of fat in your body to go down, from an average of 22 per cent in men who don't exercise to 16 per cent in those who do and from an average, for women, of 30 per cent to 20 per cent.
- It will help ensure that your blood pressure remains normal, or help to lower it if it is high.
- It will help to build up the strength of your heart so it can do its normal work effortlessly and have a bigger reserve capacity.
- It will decrease the level of cholesterol in your blood, so making less likely the build-up of fatty deposits in the arteries, which leads to strokes and heart attacks.
- In short, it will help you to become biologically younger than non-exercising people of the same age.

EXCUSES, EXCUSES

With all these benefits, taking more exercise does seem irresistible – yet so many of us do resist it, for reasons which really don't hold water.

- *I'm too fat:* Being overweight is an excellent reason to *start* exercising because it will help you to lose weight. Of course, you need to take it slowly at first but you'll soon begin to feel the benefits – and see them on your bathroom scales. If you're embarrassed about exercising with other people, begin with exercises you can do in the privacy of your own bedroom (see later in this chapter).

■ *I'm too old:*   You're never too old to exercise. Of course, as you get older you can't exercise as vigorously, but as long as you're putting in a little you're getting the maximum benefit. Regular exercise will also help to ensure a more active old age.

■ *I'm too tired:*   Regular exercise will help you to feel *less* tired. You'll find you have a lot more energy – both physical and mental – to do your everyday work and, sleeping better, you'll wake up refreshed.

■ *I feel fine:*   How you feel is a good indication of your health, but it's not the whole story. Exercise will help you to be healthy. And no matter how well you feel, you'll feel better when you exercise regularly.

■ *I'm too busy:*   If you're not used to putting aside time to exercise, you may find it difficult to fit into a busy life. But there is some form of exercise that everyone can take, however busy they are. Also you may need to assess your priorities: shouldn't being and keeping healthy be important for you? Don't think of exercise as a chore and it will become a pleasure. People who exercise regularly find that, because they're more relaxed and feel on top of things, they can cope more easily with work pressures and a busy life.

■ *I'm not sporty:*   You don't need to be: there are exercises to suit everyone. Even if you didn't enjoy playing games at school, you can find an exercise that you will enjoy. Exercise doesn't have to be competitive to be beneficial and, even in competitive exercise, you don't have to reach championship level to get the benefit from it.

Do I Need a Check-up Before I Start?

Most people, even older people, don't need a medical check-up before starting regular exercise. That we should even think of the question shows how abnormal our lives have become for exercise to be considered an esoteric, exotic, minority interest. Exercise is normal! Indeed, some American doctors – slightly tongue-in-cheek – say that you need a medical check-up if you *don't* exercise.

Obviously, if you're unfit, it's wise to take it slowly and gently at first and build up your exercise gradually. You should consult your doctor if you've suffered, or are suffering from, any of the following conditions or are worried about any other aspect of your health:

high blood pressure or heart disease
chest problems like asthma or bronchitis
back trouble or a slipped disc
joint pains or arthritis
recuperation from an illness or operation.

In all these conditions, the right exercise will help you to be healthier, but it's wise to ask your doctor's advice about the right kind of exercise for you.

If you've got a cold, flu, a sore throat or a temperature, it's wise not to exercise until you feel better.

Exercise – provided you follow the guidelines outlined in this chapter – is not dangerous. Of course, some people will have a heart attack while jogging but far more will have one lying in bed or sitting watching television, yet these are not considered dangerous pastimes! If a middle-aged person, whose arteries are already partially clogged, suddenly starts taking very vigorous exercise then he or she runs an increased risk of a heart attack. But built up gradually, exercise is not only safe, it will also help to *protect* you against having a heart attack and will improve your health in so many other ways. Someone who dies jogging might have died even earlier if he hadn't taken any exercise at all.

THE THREE 'S's OF EXERCISE

We're building up three things when we exercise: suppleness, strength and stamina.

Suppleness

We have to be able to stretch and bend and twist and turn our limbs and all our joints through a full range of movement. We need to be supple to get up and sit down, to get in and out of cars, to clean windows and even to brush our hair. As we get older, it's particularly important to try to keep our joints supple.

Strength

We need to push and pull, lift and dig. We need strength for gardening and for carrying shopping. Again, it's important to keep our muscles strong for an active old age. For all of us, strong back and stomach muscles will help to give us a good posture and help to avoid backache.

Stamina

In many ways, this is the most important thing of all. Exercise which improves stamina brings us the most benefits for our health. It's the sort of exercise which helps us to lose weight and helps to protect against heart disease. Having stamina means being able to keep going when walking quickly or when running. If we have stamina, we don't get too tired or out of breath quickly.

The best sort of exercise for stamina is aerobic exercise and it's this sort of exercise that you should start planning to build in as a permanent part of your life. It is exercise in which we're using the big muscles of the arms and legs rhythmically and where we're getting out of breath. When we do this, we're using oxygen from the air (hence 'aerobic') to release energy from our muscles. Our heart and lungs really get working and we're burning up calories.

By contrast, anaerobic exercise, like weight-lifting or taking part in a tug-of-war, requires a short, sharp burst of energy that uses a different chemical method to get our muscles to work. Although we contract our muscles in an aerobic exercise, we may not be getting out of breath.

Aerobic exercise is particularly effective when we're moving our body through space, either on land or in water. It tunes up our heart and lungs so that they're stronger and can eventually do the same work with less effort and have a greater reserve capacity.

The very best aerobic exercise for you is one you enjoy. Here are some examples to choose from:

brisk walking	energetic dancing
running or jogging	squash
swimming	running on the spot
cycling	climbing stairs
rowing	using a stationary exercise bike
tennis (especially singles)	badminton and squash.

Do it Regularly

Fitness isn't something we can store up and put away for a rainy day like money in a deposit account. We have to keep exercising throughout our lives. The ideal, for the maximum benefit to health, is to do at least a 20-minute session of exercise which gets you out of breath three times a week.

Aim for this ideal, but don't worry if you don't always achieve it – any exercise is better than nothing. But it really is worth trying to achieve it so make sure any excuses you have are not phoney either! Remember you can vary your exercise if you prefer or if it's more convenient: a couple of days a week you could do half an hour's brisk walking (perhaps split into two 15-minute segments); on another couple of days you could swim for half an hour and on another day you could play tennis for half an hour. Later in this chapter there is a detailed exercise plan for getting fit with different types of exercises.

Doing it Vigorously but Doing it Safely

To get the maximum benefit for your health your exercise should be vigorous enough to get you out of breath. You shouldn't get so out of breath that you couldn't carry on a coversation if you wanted to. And your vigorous exercise shouldn't be uncomfortable or produce pain. Stop exercising if you have any of these symptoms:

pain
dizziness
unusual fatigue
feeling sick or generally unwell.

If the symptoms persist or you're worried about them, see your doctor.

We all have a built-in monitor which tells us whether we are getting the right amount of exercise for our age and standard of physical fitness: our pulse rate, which tells us what our heart rate is. As we exercise, our heart rate goes up to supply extra oxygen to the muscles. The rate is a good guide to whether you're exercising strenuously enough or whether you're overdoing it and should slow down. The pulse rate is also a monitor of fitness: if you're unfit, you'll be able to get your heart rate up to an adequate rate just by walking.

Take your pulse by gently pressing your first two fingers of one hand on the thumb side of the other wrist or at the neck, beside the windpipe. Count how many pulses there are in 15 seconds immediately after you've exercised and then multiply it by four (to give you a rate per minute). If your pulse rate is faster than the safe maximum for your age (see table below), you need to take it more easily. If it's below the maximum rate given, then you can afford to be more vigorous. Make sure the pulse rate is at least at the minimum quoted or above it so that you're getting some benefit. You'll soon get to know what's right for you and you won't need to keep checking your pulse. If your pulse is irregular or if you have any pain in the chest as you exercise, see your doctor.

Pulse rate check

Age	Minimum per minute	Maximum per minute
20–29	140	170
30–39	130	160
40–49	125	140
50–59	115	130
60–69	105	120
70–79	95	110

START MOVING

As I've said already, if you're very unfit or if it's a long time since you took any exercise, start by increasing your physical activity slowly and gently before attempting anything vigorous. Start weaving more physical activity into your normal life. Think of ways you can start increasing your activity in all areas of your life. Write them down and keep adding to your list – and do them!

- Walk to work or to the station or at least walk part of the way.
- Walk to the shops: if you have a lot of shopping to carry back, you could get someone to come and give you a lift or return by public transport.

- Park your car some distance from your destination and walk the rest of the way.
- Think 'Can I walk there?' before using your car or getting a bus.
- Get off the bus one or two stops early and walk the rest of the way.
- Cycle to work or to the shops or just for pleasure.
- Use stairs instead of lifts or escalators whenever you can.
- Do some gardening or some *more* gardening. Mow the lawn more often.

SOMETHING MORE VIGOROUS

Once you've started to get moving, you'll want to tackle some more vigorous exercise. Brisk walking is the best one to start with but if you're under 35 and fit you may want to start with something more strenuous. Even if you're fit, however, it's always wise to take it slowly for the first five minutes as you warm up. You should start with some gentle bending and stretching exercises. Most injuries and sprains are the result of overdoing it too quickly. Always 'cool down' as well, by walking or moving slowly for a few minutes after you've finished brisk exercise. A lot of your blood is sent to your legs to supply them with oxygen during exercise. When your muscles are working hard, they help you to shift this blood back to the heart and brain. If you stop suddenly, the blood 'pools' in your legs, your brain doesn't get enough, and you may become dizzy.

After very heavy exercise, you may become dehydrated so it's wise to top up with clear fluids (which don't need to be sugary) after you've finished. If it's a hot day and you're sweating a lot perhaps drink something during exercise too.

AN EXERCISE PLAN

First decide if you're fit or unfit:

- If you're under 35 and you can run for a bus without being rendered speechless for five minutes, you can consider yourself fit. If you're over 35 and have been taking regular exercise (two or three times a week) which gets you a little breathless, you can also consider yourself fit.

- If you're over 35 and haven't had any regular exercise recently, consider yourself unfit. If you're under 35 and haven't been out of breath since you left school, then also consider yourself unfit.

As you will see, the exercise plan overleaf gives guidelines for more than 14 days. After all, the benefits of exercise build up gradually and this plan is to start you in the right direction. Try to do at least one session, three to five days a week.

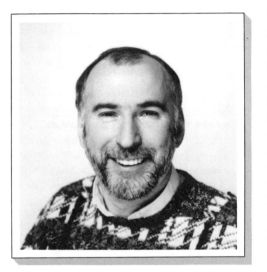

KEN BRUCE

Running for a bus recently, I was cruelly reminded that I am no longer a teenager by my utter exhaustion after a trot of only 25 yards. It's therefore no surprise that those of us approaching or hovering around the 40 mark decide to take a little exercise to try and turn back the clock. For me it's cycling – muscular effort, breathing improvements and it's less boring than jogging. Now where's that yellow jersey?

Walking

Walking is one of the very best exercises and it's an excellent way to start exercising. Walking is safe for people of all ages and it can bring you the same benefits as more vigorous forms of exercise provided you do it for long enough and walk fast enough. Aim to get out of puff.

Build up slowly and aim for a 20 to 30 minutes' walk where you get out of breath but can still carry on a normal conversation. After a while, you'll want to walk for longer as you'll feel barely warmed up after 20 minutes, so increase the length of time and try to walk part of the way uphill.

SUGGESTIONS FOR AN EXERCISE PLAN - DO THREE TO FIVE SESSIONS PER WEEK

		Week 1 Minutes per session	Week 2	
Brisk Walking	Unfit	10	15	
	Fit	15	20	
Swimming	Unfit	5	10	
(continuous)	Fit	10	15	
Skipping	Unfit	3	4	
	Fit	7	10	
Rowing &	Unfit	5	7	
Cycling Machine	Fit	10	12	
Aerobics Dancing	Unfit	5	8	
	Fit	20	25	
Cycling	Unfit	5	7	
	Fit	15	20	
Jogging	Unfit	Don't jog – 10 mins brisk walking	10 mins brisk walk & 2 mins jog & 3 mins brisk walk	
	Fit	10 mins brisk walk & 4 mins jog & 6 mins brisk walk	10 mins brisk walk & 6 mins jog & 4 mins brisk walk	

Swimming

This is probably the ideal all-round exercise. It's excellent for stamina, strength and suppleness. It's good for people of all ages and all levels of physical fitness. It's especially good if you have joint problems or backache, or if you're overweight, as the water supports the weight of your body. It's something you can do with all the family, too, but splashing around at the shallow end with the kids doesn't count as aerobic exercise. To get the maximum benefit you need to swim laps using one of the serious strokes: crawl, butterfly, backstroke or breast-stroke. Build up your stamina to the point where you can swim for 20 minutes without stopping.

Week 3	Week 4	Week 5	Week 6
20	25	30	35
25	30	35	40
15	20	25	30
20	25	30	35
5	6	7	8
12	15	17	20
10	12	15	20
15	20	25	30
10	12	15	20
30	30	30	30
10	15	20	25
25	30	35	40
10 mins brisk walk & 4 mins jog & 6 mins brisk walk	10 mins brisk walk & 6 mins jog & 4 mins brisk walk	10 mins brisk walk & 8 mins jog & 7 mins brisk walk	10 mins brisk walk & 10 mins jog & 5 mins brisk walk
5 mins brisk walk & 8 mins jog & 5 mins brisk walk & 4 mins jog & 2 mins brisk walk	5 mins brisk walk & 10 mins jog & 5 mins brisk walk & 5 mins jog & 2 mins brisk walk	5 mins brisk walk & 12 mins jog & 4 mins rest & 6 mins jog & 5 mins brisk walk	5 mins brisk walk & 15 mins jog & 5 mins brisk walk & 10 mins jog & 5 mins brisk walk

Skipping and indoor stationary machines

If you don't want to get out of breath in public and prefer to exercise at home, or if you are too busy to go out to exercise, you can still get fit. Skipping with a rope or running on the spot will provide you with aerobic exercise. You may find it boring, but you could always listen to music at the same time. Repeatedly going up and down stairs will give you aerobic exercise too. You need to take this easy, though, as it can very quickly raise your heart rate, so check your pulse. Stepping on and off a bench or block 9–12 inches high will give you the same sort of beneficial exercise.

Stationary bikes and rowing machines will also give you good aerobic exercise. The best kinds of exercise bikes have adjustable resistance on the pedals that you can work harder as you get fitter.

Both bikes and rowing machines are excellent for getting and keeping fit. Again, the problem may be boredom. But you can watch television, listen to the radio, read, or have a conversation at the same time. This may be the solution if you have a very busy life and can't see where exercise would fit into it. They're expensive to buy, though, so be sure you're going to use them before you do splash out.

Dancing

Waltzing isn't going to do too much for your health, though vigorous disco dancing may provide aerobic exercise. Aerobic dancing classes, however, do provide a way of getting exercise which really is of benefit. Some of them have been criticised for pushing people too quickly and so causing them injuries or sprains, but some people enjoy exercising in company and find it encourages them to keep going. If you begin gradually, aerobics classes are a good way of getting exercise. Dancing is excellent for strength in your leg muscles, good for stamina and helps to keep your joints supple.

Cycling

This is good for stamina and for strength in the leg muscles. It will help with suppleness as you get older. Again, cycling may be a pleasant pastime for the whole family. To ensure you get aerobic exercise, though, you have to get your legs moving hard and rhythmically. Make sure you know your Highway Code and wear reflective clothing at night.

Running or jogging

These are really the same thing: a jog is a slow run. Jogging is very good for stamina but not so good for suppleness and strength (apart from your leg muscles). You can run at whatever speed suits you and it will increase your level of fitness quickly and efficiently. Again, you need to go slowly for several months, at first alternately jogging and walking. Build up gradually and don't get too out of breath. You're not in a race, so don't increase your speed until you're ready. The time you spend jogging is more important than the speed you jog at.

Try to run on grass whenever you can as it's easier on your feet. You do need to buy a good pair of running shoes: go to a specialist shop and ask for advice. You'll get a lot of advice and help, too, if you join an athletics club. Jogging with a friend will also encourage you to do it on a regular basis and not to skip it if you don't feel like it on a particular day.

Badminton, tennis, and squash

Badminton and tennis can be fun to play even if you're a beginner, but the benefit to your health increases as your play improves. Then the exercise each provides becomes more aerobic, with fewer stops and starts. Singles tennis is likely to be more vigorous than doubles and so more beneficial. Again, both can be family games.

You should already be fit when you start playing squash; it can be a fast and hard game, but it is excellent for stamina. If you're over 35 when you start, make sure you begin by playing very gently.

Other games

Judge whether other games will help your stamina by considering if they get your large muscles moving rhythmically over a period of time, getting breathless in the process. Obviously, rugby and soccer do (unless you're in goal) while cricket does not. Golf is a decent exercise if you carry your own clubs and walk fast, but it's unlikely to provide you with a vigorous exercise. Like bowls, it helps to keep you supple as you get older.

Keep At It

Remember, you don't need to keep to just one form of exercise: you can ring the changes. Remember, too, that you can't keep exercise on deposit – it has to be like a hard working current account! But once you start to exercise regularly, you'll enjoy it so much and feel so much benefit from it, that you'll wonder why you didn't always do it.

4 IS IT WORTH ONE MORE PUFF? STOP SMOKING WITH THE 14-DAY PLAN

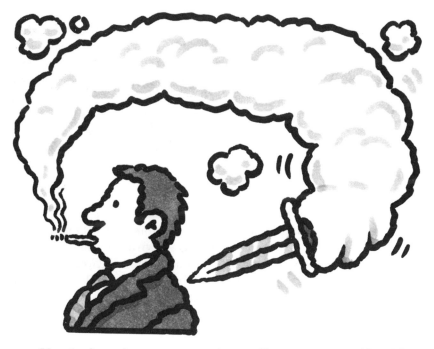

You don't need me or anyone else to tell you to stop smoking. Most smokers want to stop. But before you do it, you yourself need to make the definite *decision* that you want to stop now. This chapter will help you to make that decision by telling you how risky it is, but more importantly, it will also tell you how you can motivate yourself and maximise your own will power to enable you to succeed in stopping and to keep stopped. Ten million people in Britain have stopped smoking and you can join them. Have the confidence you can do it: you can.

Everyone who smokes knows that it's dangerous. On every cigarette packet, on every magazine advert, on every advertising hoarding you can see the message: 'Smoking can seriously damage your health'. To try to jolt the complacent there are now some even more graphic messages. All of them are true, but the truest one of all isn't there: SMOKING KILLS.

If everyone who smokes knows that it's dangerous, how many know just *how* dangerous? For every 1,000 young men who smoke, 250 will be killed before their time – usually in their forties or fifties – by cigarettes they say are a pleasure, a relaxation. Some pleasure! Some relaxation! It's like dodging traffic on motorways for a hobby or playing Russian roulette with one live bullet for every three dummies. Remember that there's no safe level of smoking. Even two or three cigarettes per day increase your risk of fatal diseases.

Cancer is the second biggest cause of death in this country. Lung cancer is the most common cancer amongst men and well over 90 per cent of lung cancer is caused by smoking. Regular smokers are up to 40 times more likely to develop lung cancer than non-smokers. Amongst women breast cancer has, up until now, been the most common cancer but now lung cancer is overtaking it. Fewer numbers of women have stopped smoking compared with men and, what is particularly worrying, young women are smoking more.

The biggest cause of death in Britain is heart disease. Although lung cancer is so strongly associated in everyone's mind with smoking – and getting on for 40,000 smokers die every year from lung cancer – many more smokers die of a heart attack. At least 20 per cent of heart attacks are attributable to smoking. For men between the ages of 30 and 59, smoking 20 cigarettes a day or more *trebles* the risk of heart attack. Smoking 40 cigarettes a day increases the risk of heart disease by *20 times*.

As well as these common ways that smoking kills vast numbers of people every day, smoking is implicated too in cancer of the mouth, of the throat, of the voice box or larynx and of the food-pipe or oesophagus. It can also cause other unpleasant lung diseases like bronchitis or emphysema, which is a disease where the internal structure of the lung breaks down. A victim of either of these diseases can be so disabled that he or she can't walk from one side of the room to the other without becoming breathless.

The first link between smoking and lung cancer was made in 1948 and that between smoking and heart disease in 1951. As evidence pointing to the association between smoking and these killer diseases became stronger and stronger, doctors in Britain began to stop smoking in large numbers. As they did so, their death rate began to fall compared with other British men of the same age. All over the world, the same result was seen: when people gave up smoking, they began to live longer than smokers.

If you ask any doctor he or she will tell you that nearly *everyone* gives up smoking when told they have lung cancer or after a heart attack. Why don't you kick the habit now before it kicks you? The good news is that a smoker who stops smoking reduces the risk of lung cancer over a period of time and from day one reduces the risk of a heart attack. After a few years, the risk of a heart attack is almost down to what it would have been if he or she had always been a non-smoker (see Chapter 6).

WOMEN AND SMOKING

Much of the research into smoking refers to men because, in the past, they tended to smoke much more than women did. Consequently, lung cancer was more common amongst men. In addition to this, because of their smoking as well as the fact that being male in itself is a factor, men are more likely to have a heart attack in middle age than women. But over the last 15 years in Britain, rates of heart disease have risen faster in women than in men and lung cancer is now overtaking breast cancer as the most common cancer amongst women.

The reason for the increase is that women are smoking more cigarettes than they used to. Although fewer women are smoking overall, the number of teenage girls who smoke is going up and those who do smoke are smoking more. The risk of lung cancer increases with the number of cigarettes smoked.

It also appears that smoking may bring on an earlier menopause and so cause women to lose the protection that their hormones give them against having a heart attack (see page 91). If older women who are using oral contraception (the 'Pill') smoke, then they dangerously increase their risk of a heart attack (see page 92).

Women also have another very important reason not to smoke. Babies born to women who smoke tend to have lower birth weights and there are some indications that this retarded growth in the womb may continue to affect children as they grow up. Babies of mothers who smoke are more likely to develop pneumonia in the first year of life.

STILL NOT CONVINCED?

Remember that rather than try to convince you that you should stop smoking, I'm aiming to help you to come to that inner certainty so that you can say with conviction 'Yes, I want to stop smoking now'. As you're struggling with yourself, you may find that several excuses drift into your mind. Let's look at them.

■ *I'll lose my only pleasure in life:* I'm sure, no matter how much you enjoy smoking, that it isn't your *only* pleasure in life. In your heart, you know this excuse is phoney – ask a friend who's given up smoking. When you stop you'll feel fitter and fresher and won't want to go back to the dubious 'pleasure' of cigarettes. Just think of all the new pleasures you'll be able to afford with the money you save.

■ *I'll be impossible to live with:* It's true that some people do get edgy and irritable when they give up smoking, but it usually passes off very quickly. Anyway, think of what you're inflicting on your family and friends by forcing them to inhale your second-hand cigarette smoke. They'll bear a few days of your being grumpy if it means – as it will – that you're going to be healthier and live longer.

■ *I've given up before and I got a cough and sore-throat:* It's not surprising that some people develop a cough *after* they give up smoking. Coughing is a natural reaction: it means that your lungs' defence systems are beginning to work again. They'd quite literally been paralysed by cigarette smoke and now they are beginning to bring up all the muck that's been deposited in them when you were smoking. If you get a sore throat after stopping that's understand-able too: cigarette smoke irritates your throat but it also numbs it. So a slight discomfort means that your throat is returning to normal.

- *I'll put on weight:* It's an absolute myth that *everyone* who stops smoking puts on weight though it's true that some people do. Even if you did put on some extra weight, though, it would be a very small risk to your health compared with the risks of smoking. In fact you'd have to put on 10 stone to equal the risk of smoking 20 cigarettes a day! But you don't need to put on any weight at all if you follow the guidelines in Chapters 1 and 2 on healthy eating and losing weight. And taking exercise is going to stop you putting on weight too (see Chapter 3).
- *I've got to die of something:* Sure – but when? Do you want to have the very best chance of reaching three score years and ten or do you want instead to give yourself the best possible chance of dying in middle age of lung cancer or a heart attack? Remember, even if you don't die of one of these diseases, you could end up living a life of breathless misery.

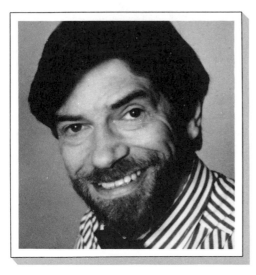

ADRIAN LOVE

I smoke 60 cigarettes a day and have smoked for about 28 years. I can't say I enjoy smoking – but I enjoy *not* smoking less. I've tried to give up several times before. The longest time I stopped was when I heard a good friend had cancer; I came home, threw all my cigarettes in the house away (about 200 – I'd just come back from abroad). I broke them all up and poured water over them and then I didn't smoke for nine days. Then at a party I suddenly noticed I had a half-smoked cigarette in my hand – it was totally unconscious. I really do want to give up now – my family is so keen that I stop. I think the advice I'd give to anyone, which I'm going to take myself, is not to have any cigarettes in the house; to tell everyone you know you're going to stop smoking and ask them to help; and to be really on your guard that you're not tempted by 'just' one cigarette.

We all know of the apocryphal figure who smoked 40 cigarettes a day and lived till he was 90. Some people do take risks like that and get away with it, but they are very few and far between. Most of us are extremely susceptible to the risks of smoking. After all, 90-year-old smokers are a great rarity; victims of heart attacks and lung cancer in their forties and fifties are tragically common.

14-DAY PLAN FOR STOPPING SMOKING:

The decision

Remember your personal decision to stop is crucial. Being convinced in your own mind that you do want to stop is the best foundation for success. This 14-day plan tells you how to build on that foundation. If you're not yet convinced (remember: don't rely on what other people tell you or even what you tell them) then go through the preparation steps in Days 1 to 6. That should convince you why you want to stop. If you haven't decided, don't go on to Day 7 and stop, but go back to Day 1 and start again. Don't go to Day 7 half-heartedly because you'll then have less chance of success; if you don't succeed you may start to try to convince yourself that you knew all along that you could never give up smoking. You can.

Preparation

As in losing weight, preparation is the key to success in giving up smoking. You'll be mobilising every physical and mental faculty in your make-up to help you to succeed. That's why the first half of the 14-day plan is preparing: you only stop smoking on Day 7. Even if you're desperate to stop straight away, you're more likely to succeed in the long term if you choose that day a week away as a stop-day and lead up to it, like an athlete in training.

If you're convinced you want to stop but are dreading actually doing it, remember I'm not asking you to give up now but to carry on smoking for one final week and then, much better prepared, I assure you you'll find it easier to stop. Remember that preparation days are designed to help you use all the tricks in the book to help you achieve your goal. Even if you feel that some of them are not for you, do try them all. You're going to battle and you may as well have every weapon at hand you can.

SMOKING DIARY   Day **MONDAY**

Time	What were you doing?	Who were you with?
7.30 am	Having breakfast	Alone
8.30 am	Opening letters in the office	Anne and Sue
9.15 am	Typing	Anne and Sue
10.40 am	Having coffee	Joan
10.50 am	Talking	Joan
11.10 am	Typing	In office with Anne and Sue
11.20 am	Typing	
11.40 am	Typing	

Day 1

- Keep a 'smoking diary' for the next week. Get a notebook to keep the diary and also to write down the other things I'll be asking you to do in the next week. Write down the time and circumstances of every cigarette you smoke. There's an example of how a smoking diary might look above.

  Once you've kept it for a few days, you should start asking yourself some questions about it.

How were you feeling?	How much did you enjoy it?	How much did you need it?
Tired	Not a lot	A lot
Relaxed	Not much	Not much
Busy	A little	Not very much
} Feeling relaxed	A great deal	Quite a bit
	Quite a lot	Not at all
Feeling under pressure to finish this report by lunchtime	Not at all	A little
	Not really	Quite a lot
	Hardly at all	A great deal

What sort of activities provoke me into having a cigarette? (For example, do I *always* smoke while having a coffee?)

Who provokes me into having a cigarette? (For example, do I *always* have one when I chat to Sue?)

Which cigarettes did I find most enjoyable and why?

Which cigarettes could I easily have not smoked and why?

Which cigarettes did I feel I could not have done without and why?

The information you find out about your smoking habits is going to be very useful to you when you stop. You've highlighted the problem areas and so you're halfway to tackling them and taking avoidance action when temptation creeps in. You may find, incidentally, that just the act of writing it down in your diary each time you smoke causes you to cut down the number of cigarettes you get through. Don't worry if it doesn't, but if it does it's a useful bonus.

■ Get a glass jar and start collecting all your cigarette ends in it. When you're out or at work, keep them in an empty cigarette packet and then add them to the jar when you get home. Look at the cigarette ends in the jar when you smoke.

Day 2

■ Write down, preferably in your notebook, your reasons for wanting to stop smoking. Try to think of as many reasons as possible that are important to you. Don't worry if some of the reasons are rather silly – this is a private list and you don't need to show it to anybody. Try to think of at least 10. You'll probably find that your own personal reasons are more important than general or 'medical' reasons. (Though those reasons are very important as well!) You're trying here to find a strong motivation to stop smoking – to help increase your will power when you stop – and so the most powerful reasons for this purpose will be the ones that you yourself think are important. Your list might look something like this:

'My husband/wife wants me to stop.'
'I know my children would be delighted if I stopped.'
'I'd have more money to spend on clothes.'
'I'd feel I'd be in control of my own body.'
'I want to feel my breath doesn't smell.'
'I'd feel sexier if I stopped.'
'I want to be able to play with my children without getting out of breath.'
'I resent giving the Chancellor all those hard-earned pounds.'
'I don't want to come down in the morning to the smell of stale cigarette smoke.'

Have a really good think and write down your own reasons. Keep the list and add to it if you can over the coming days.

- Start changing brands. Each time you buy a packet of cigarettes, try to get a different brand, preferably milder, lower-tar cigarettes. This will make it that much easier when you do come to stop.

Day 3

- Tell all your family and friends that you're going to stop in a few days' time. This should have two beneficial effects: you'll feel you have committed yourself and that will further strengthen your resolve; you'll find that most of your friends will be encouraging and will help you even if it's only by kind words and sympathy. Tell them how really important it is for you to stop and how much you'd appreciate their support when you stop. You may find friends who are ex-smokers particularly helpful; smoking friends may scoff (but remember that in their heart they probably want to give up too).
- Put two elastic bands around each cigarette packet you buy and keep them there. The mere act of having to take the bands off is going to make you think about every cigarette you smoke. Very often, I'm sure, you reach for a cigarette without knowing you're doing it. I'm not telling you to cut down the number of cigarettes you smoke, but you should ask yourself each time you undo the elastic bands 'Do I really want, do I really need, this cigarette?' Again, you may find that, without trying, you have cut down the number of cigarettes you smoke.

Day 4

- Calculate and write down the money you spend on cigarettes each day, each week, each month, each year.
- Think of some treats you'd really like to buy yourself with the sort of sums you spend on cigarettes. Write down as many as you can think of. They'll range, perhaps, from a bunch of daffodils to a holiday in Majorca, or from a cassette to a CD sound system.
- Stop carrying a lighter or matches so that you'll have to make yet another conscious effort to have a cigarette.

Day 5

- Tell all the smokers you're likely to meet at work or socially that it's really important not to offer you a cigarette from now on. Tell them you're going to stop in two days.
- Start concentrating completely on every single cigarette you smoke. As you smoke don't do anything else at all – don't talk, don't drink, don't read, don't watch TV or listen to the radio. Smoke each cigarette quickly and concentrate on your senses, your sense of taste and your sense of smell. Think about the effect each cigarette is having on your body: the smoke and tar going down into your lungs, the nicotine and carbon monoxide (both deadly poisonous) going into your bloodstream.

Day 6

- Read through your smoking diary. Note the difficult situations when you always have a cigarette and begin to think what you are going to do about them. For example, if you always have a cigarette with coffee, cut out the coffee or have fruit juice or milk instead. Note which are your 'key' cigarettes – the ones you really enjoy or feel you need. Those are the times when you're really going to have to be on your guard.
- Look again at your calculations of the money you're going to save. Start imagining the treats you're going to buy for yourself out of the money you've spent up until now on your cigarettes.

Day 7: Stop day

- As soon as you wake up today, say to yourself 'I don't want to smoke'.
- Get another glass jar and start putting into it all the money you would have spent on cigarettes.
- Be alert for those times of the day when you know you'll be vulnerable to the temptation to smoke.
- Give yourself a treat. Buy yourself something or go out for a meal (but don't reach for a cigarette after your food).

Day 8

- When you wake up say, 'I am now a non-smoker'. You've now gone a day without cigarettes. Congratulate yourself. You're going to take one day at a time, but if you've done one day, you can do another and another.
- Watch out for withdrawal symptoms. You may get sleepy or become restless and irritable. But remember that many people get no withdrawal symptoms at all.
- Avoid situations which may tempt you to smoke. For example, if you always smoke at the end of a meal, get up from the table straight away.

Day 9

- When you wake up, practise saying, 'No, thanks, I don't smoke, no thanks I don't smoke'. Soon it will become an instant automatic response if someone offers you a cigarette.
- If you get a craving for a cigarette, tell yourself that *you're* in control now, not the nicotine. Time the craving: you'll find it will only last a few minutes. The act of timing it gives you power over it.
- If you get a very strong urge to smoke, deal with it by doing something: take a quick walk, do some gardening, chew a pencil, eat an apple or a carrot, chew some gum, brush your teeth or take a shower. Think of your own variations. By the time you've taken some diverting action like this, the urge to smoke will have passed.

Day 10

- When you wake up, look again at all the reasons for stopping that you've written down. Add to them if you can.
- Think of other ways of resisting the urge to smoke. Deep breathing works for many people. Take a big breath and then breathe out very slowly, saying to yourself 'I do not want to smoke', as you do so.
- Keep looking at the jar into which you're putting the money you're saving.

Day 11

- When you wake up, tell yourself you've now gone four days without smoking. You're succeeding, you're now a non-smoker.
- List all the advantages you can think of that you've gained by being a non-smoker.
- If you're feeling tense and unrelaxed, look at Chapter 8 and choose one of the methods suggested there to help you relax.

Day 12

- Remind yourself that you're taking one day at a time. As each day goes by without a cigarette, you're building up an investment. Tell yourself you're not going to throw it away.
- Think of beginning to take some regular exercise. You can really start to get fit and it's a very good diversion from temptation. Exercise is also a very good way of relaxing. See Chapter 3 for some suggestions.
- Look again at your savings jar. Look at your calculations of how much you're going to save in a month and a year and think again of how you're going to spend the money.

Day 13

- Make sure you're not tempted to accept 'just' one cigarette from someone. One leads to another and another.
- Keep adding to your list of advantages of being a non-smoker.

    My breath smells fresher.
    I can taste my food more.
    My clothes don't smell of stale tobacco smoke.
    I'm in charge of my own body.

- For a few weeks, if possible, avoid social situations where you smoked. When you've had a few drinks, you'll be an easy prey for the temptation to have a cigarette.

Day 14

- When you wake up, remind yourself that you've now been a non-smoker for a whole week. Congratulate yourself. If you can go one week without smoking, you can go one month, one year, one whole lifetime.
- Buy yourself something nice. Remember you're rewarding yourself – you really have achieved something.
- Read through again your reasons for stopping and keep thinking of them in the coming days.

STAYING STOPPED

- Be on your guard. Remember all the tricks you've learnt about how to overcome temptation.
- Even after a year, you could get hooked again. Beware of accepting even *one* cigarette. Don't be complacent because you've succeeded – that one cigarette could take you back along the road to smoking.
- One month, and then one year, after you've stopped buy yourself something with the money you've saved.

FAILURE PAVES THE WAY TO SUCCESS

- If you do have one cigarette, don't feel you've failed. Think of how you're going to resist the temptation next time.
- If you do go back to smoking, as soon as you can make that decision to stop again.
- Start the 14-day plan again as soon as you can. You'll know quite a bit about how you'll stop it happening again. Though you've lost one battle, be determined to win the war.
- Two-thirds of ex-smokers say they found it easy to stop, but some people do find it difficult. Everyone can do it though. Remember that ten million people in Britain are ex-smokers and many of them gave up more than once before they finally succeeded.

OTHER WAYS OF GETTING HELP

- People find many different ways useful and helpful in stopping smoking: our 14-day plan is just one reliable and tested way of stopping.

- Acupuncture and hypnosis help some people, although the snag is you'll probably have to pay for them.
- Ask your GP for advice. He or she may refer you to a stop-smoking course in the area. If you're lucky, your general practice may run courses itself. Your GP will also give encouragement and advice and may decide to prescribe nicotine chewing-gum. This has been shown to be effective in helping people to stop smoking. Unfortunately, it's not available on an NHS prescription, so you'll have to pay the full price for it – but it's much cheaper than smoking.
- Don't waste your money on advertised 'magic' cures to stop smoking. Take the advice of your own doctor.
- In the end, it comes back to your own will power and motivation. We've seen in this chapter how you can harness and strengthen these. You don't need an extraordinary iron will to succeed, but you do need to be determined and to make that definite decision to give up. Then you'll do it.

5 DRINKING ALCOHOL SENSIBLY

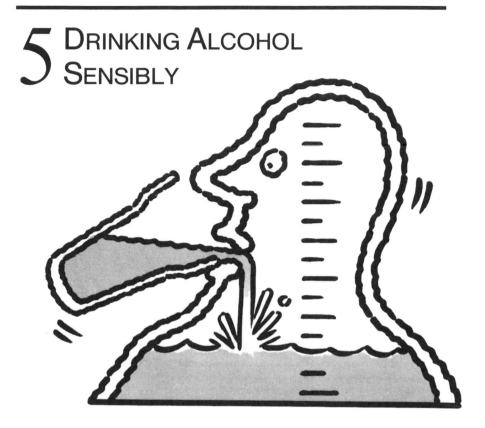

'Wine gladdens the heart of man', as the Bible puts it. Alcohol is certainly a great pleasure. It is the most widely used recreational drug and if we're sensible alcohol is enjoyable and may even do us some good. But, like any drug, alcohol can be misused. We can, of course, drink too much of it, both in the short term and the long term. We can drink it in inappropriate situations, like before driving or before operating machinery. And *misusing* alcohol can do a great deal of harm to our health or even kill us.

The medical advice about drinking is not the same as the medical advice about smoking, which is, of course, don't do it. It is possible to go on drinking and enjoying alcohol but in a way which is safe and doesn't endanger your health and life, nor indeed the lives of others.

WHAT'S THE PROBLEM?

The problem of alcohol misuse is not new. In 1726, the Royal College of Physicians (in a report to the House of Commons) said of drinking in excess: 'this custom doth every year increase, notwithstanding our repeated advices to the contrary... [it is] a great and growing evil.' Two hundred and sixty years later, the Royal College of Physicians wrote another report on the increasing numbers of patients damaged by alcohol. It states that about one in five of all men admitted to hospital medical wards has a problem related to alcohol abuse.

So, it's obvious that the problems associated with alcohol are not confined to those on 'skid row' or those who could be considered alcoholics. Very large numbers of people in this country are drinking in quantities which will damage their health and all of us who drink need to consider whether or not we're drinking within safe limits.

HOW MUCH DO WE DRINK?

Alcohol consumption has risen sharply in the UK in the last 30 years after falling consistently from the beginning of the century to the Second World War. During the last decade, beer consumption has been at its highest level for 60 years; in the past 20 years, consumption of spirits has more than doubled, and wine consumption has quadrupled.

Death rates from cirrhosis of the liver, which is caused by alcohol, have paralleled these increased alcohol consumption rates. From 1950 onwards there has been an increase in deaths from this cause.

In 1983, the average annual consumption of alcoholic drinks per person aged 15 or over was 243 pints (138 litres) of beer, 16 bottles (12 litres) of wine, 12 pints (7 litres) of cider and 7 bottles (5 litres) of spirits like whisky and gin. That's an enormous quantity of booze – and doesn't include home-brewed beer and wine. On average, men drink twice as much as women. It's true that we don't drink as much in this country as in some European countries like Germany, France and Spain but then we don't have their very high death rates for cirrhosis of the liver either.

What Happens When We Drink?

We usually think of drink as a stimulant – it makes many people more talkative and funny. But it makes others silent and withdrawn and, in fact, alcohol acts on all of us not as a stimulant but as a depressant.

Most of the alcohol we drink is absorbed by our blood stream. It's mostly processed into energy by the liver, but a small part of it is excreted in the sweat and urine. The concentration of alcohol in the body depends on whether we are male or female (see p. 80), how heavy we are, how tall we are and whether or not we're drinking on an empty stomach. 'It's gone to my head' is quite literally true. On an empty stomach, alcohol is easily absorbed into the bloodstream and is soon sloshing about the brain. Alcohol dulls the working of the brain and makes it work less efficiently. It particularly quickly affects co-ordination skills – the sort of skills we need for drinking without spilling any!

When you've drunk too much, the only thing that can sober you up is time – the time it takes for the liver to burn up the quantity of alcohol you've drunk. This may take many hours (see p. 84). Cold showers, fresh air and black coffee – or indeed anything else – have no effect whatsoever on the concentration of alcohol in your body or in your brain.

What is Safe Drinking?

There is a level of drinking below which doctors are pretty sure you're not doing any damage to your health. If you drink above this level, drinking may start becoming a hazard and, if you go further and further above this safe level, drinking does become definitely dangerous.

The problem is: what's the safe level? As we drink such a wide range of drinks – beer, lager, spirits and wine – we have to have some means of comparing these drinks with each other. It's possible to convert every drink you have into 'units' of alcohol and it's very easy to calculate this. The following are each equivalent to one 'unit':   ½ pint beer
½ pint lager
1 glass of sherry *or* martini
1 small glass red *or* white table wine
1 single gin *or* whisky (or other spirit).

There are some surprises in this list. You'll see that 1 glass of wine is equal to ½ pint of beer, so of course 2 glasses of wine equals 1 pint of beer. One pint of beer also equals a double measure of spirits like whisky. One of the commonest mistakes people make is underestimating the strength of beer: there's a mistaken belief that if you just stick to beer, you can't do yourself any harm. Opposite is a more detailed table showing how many units there are in each type of drink. Remember that these figures are approximate.

One last thing to note is that these are pub measures – a smallish glass of wine therefore. Of course, we all know how little a pub measure of spirits looks. If we were pouring one at home, we might easily give ourselves triple this quantity – and that would be three units of alcohol.

Now here's the interesting part: how many units of alcohol do you drink a week? Don't just guess at it – you'd be surprised how wrong people can be when they try to guess. What you need to do is fill in a chart with a typical week's drinking. There's a chart on pp. 78–9. Do it now by filling in what you had to drink last week. Go through each day in your mind, remembering where you were and what you were doing.

Do be honest with yourself – remember this chart is only to help you and you don't need to show it to anyone. Don't try to kid yourself that last week wasn't typical, unless it really was the sort of unusual week that happens only every five years!

A more accurate way of assessing your own drinking is to keep a chart for next week and fill it in every day – though it is possible that the act of writing down your drinking may in itself cause you to cut down. If you can, do both last week *and* next week and then you'll get a better idea of how many units you are drinking every week. Now see where your total number of units in the week puts you on the safety spectrum.

Type of Drink	Amount	Units
Beers and Lagers		
ordinary strength beer *or* lager	½ pint	1
	1 pint	2
	1 can	1½
export beer	1 pint	2½
	1 can	2
strong ale *or* lager	½ pint	2
	1 pint	4
	1 can	3
extra-strength beer *or* lager	½ pint	2½
	1 pint	5
	1 can	4
Ciders		
average cider	½ pint	1½
	1 pint	3
	quart bottle	6
strong cider	½ pint	2
	1 pint	4
	quart bottle	8
Spirits		
like whisky, gin, vodka *or* rum	1 standard single measure in most of England and Wales (⅙ gill)	1
	⅕ gill measure	1¼
	1 standard single measure in N. Ireland and some parts of Scotland (¼ gill)	1½
	1 bottle	30
Table wine		
	1 standard glass	1
	1 bottle	7
	1 litre bottle	10
Sherry, Port and Fortified Wine (like Martinis and Vermouth)		
	1 standard small measure	1
	1 bottle	12

How Many Units Of Alcohol Do You Drink In A Week?

Day	When	Where
Friday	Morning Afternoon Evening	— In office At home
Saturday	Morning Afternoon Evening	— In pub In restaurant
Sunday	Morning Afternoon Evening	In pub At home At Liz + Tony's house
Monday	Morning Afternoon Evening	— — At home
Tuesday	Morning Afternoon Evening	— — At home
Wednesday	Morning Afternoon Evening	— In pub In pub
Thursday	Morning Afternoon Evening	— At home In pub

Men	Women
Up to 21 units a week	Up to 14 units a week

Congratulations! This is sensible and safe drinking. Try to ensure your drinking is spread evenly throughout the week. (This level is not completely safe for pregnant women though – see pp. 82–3.)

With whom	What	Units	Total for day
Whole department My wife	2 glasses red wine 1 gin+Tonic, 3 glasses red wine	2 1 3	6
Bob + John My wife	2 pints beer 2 G+Ts 3 Glasses white wine	4 2 3	9
Bob + John My wife With them + my wife	2 pints beer 1 Sherry - 2 red wine 3 white wine, 1 Large whisky	4 3 3 1	11
My wife	1 red wine	1	1
My wife	2 cans lager	3	3
Clients Clients	1 pint of beer 1 G+T, 3 red wine	2 4	6
My wife Bob + John	2 white wine 2 pints beer	2 4	6

Total units for week **42**

Men	Women
22–35 units a week	15–21 units a week

You're beginning to drink too much. Try to start cutting down, which you should be able to do fairly easily.

Men	Women
36–49 units a week	22–35 units a week

At this level, damage to health is likely. You may also be getting into problems at work or at home because of your drinking. Cut down now. If there are one or two particular days when you drink heavily, concentrate on cutting down drinking then.

Men	Women
50 or more units a week	36 or more units a week

It's extremely likely that you're seriously damaging your health. This is really unsafe drinking. Start cutting down now (see p. 84). If you find you can't cut down, you really need some professional help (see pp. 141–2). You may already be dependent on alcohol without realising it.

It does seem unfair that the safe limits for men are higher than those for women – but it's not prejudice, it's physiology. The composition of women's bodies compared with men's is higher in fat but lower in water. As alcohol is distributed through the body's fluids – that is, the body's water content – the same amount of alcohol is 'diluted' more in men than it is in women. Also, a woman's liver is more susceptible than a man's to the damage that alcohol does to it. That certainly doesn't mean that a male liver is immune of course!

Sensible Drinking Guidelines

For men	For women
Up to 21 units, spread throughout the week. It's wise to have two or three days without alcohol at all.	Up to 14 units, spread throughout the week. It's wise to have two or three days without alcohol at all.

- Having two or three alcohol-free days a week allows your body to recover from the effects of alcohol.
- Remember that there are times when one or two drinks can be too much – like before driving or operating machinery.
- Always consult your doctor about drinking while taking any tablets or medicines – the combination of these and alcohol may be dangerous.

■ If you're drinking beyond these sensible guidelines see p. 84 for advice on how to cut down. There are many reasons why you should do so.

WHAT ARE THE RISKS OF UNSAFE DRINKING?

Heavy drinkers increase their risk of a wide range of diseases compared with light drinkers and non-drinkers. Alcohol can affect many different organs in the body and not just the liver. Let's take a look at the effects of heavy drinking:

On the heart

Heavy drinkers are twice as likely to die of heart disease. Long-term heavy alcohol intake can damage the heart muscle (alcoholic cardiomyopathy) which can lead to heart failure and death.

On blood pressure

Alcohol tends to increase blood pressure in susceptible people (see Chapter 7). Very heavy drinking sessions can precipitate strokes in young adults.

On cancer rates

Heavy drinkers are twice as likely to die of cancer (see p. 124). With some cancers – like those of the mouth and gullet – the risk is increased tenfold.

On the liver

Heavy drinkers are 12 times more likely to die of cirrhosis of the liver, a condition characterised by scarring of the liver.

On the pancreas

The pancreas gland can become inflamed in heavy drinkers leading to diabetes in some and preventing the proper absorption of food.

On the nervous system

Heavy drinking can cause brain haemorrhages, brain damage and dementia. It can also cause weakness and paralysis in the arms and legs and burning sensations in the hands and feet.

On men

As Shakespeare put it in *Macbeth*, alcohol 'provokes the desire but takes away the performance.' 'Brewer's droop' is of course a well-recognised immediate consequence of drinking too much alcohol. However, in the long term heavy drinkers can experience the loss of sexual desire, impotence, reduced fertility, loss of sexual hair and shrinkage in the size of the penis and testes. So much for the macho image of a great deal of the alcohol advertising around. There's one place that all beers seem to be able to reach!

On women

Similarly, heavy drinking affects women's sexual functioning, causing menstrual problems like irregular or infrequent periods; shrinkage of breasts, ovaries and external genitalia; and a progressive defeminisation with sexual difficulties and loss of vaginal secretions.

Apart from the increased difficulty in getting pregnant in the first place, women who drink heavily double their risk of having a miscarriage if they do get pregnant.

On unborn babies

Most importantly of all, women who drink alcohol during pregnancy run the risk of doing damage to their unborn baby. Obviously, the greatest risk is for women who drink heavily. Heavy drinking (about 6 units a day) can have a very severe effect on the baby leading to abnormal facial features and mental retardation. From conception onwards the less you drink, the better your chances of a normal pregnancy and a healthy baby. In fact, it seems that it's wise to cut down your drinking *before* you get pregnant. If you do drink a small amount of alcohol occasionally, the risk to your baby will be small but even moderate drinking may lead to babies of low birth weight who continue to be smaller than babies of the same age. If you don't drink alcohol at all while you're pregnant then you cut out this risk completely.

When a pregnant woman does drink, the alcohol, which is a small molecule, passes easily through the placenta and into the baby's bloodstream. Like any other drug or chemical, alcohol may damage the baby in three ways:

- by damaging the genetic material in the cells in the early phases when the fertilised egg is dividing
- by interfering with organ formation at the embryo stage (16–24 days old) and causing structural abnormalities
- by restricting the development of rapidly growing tissues, especially the brain (when the baby is 73–280 days old).

Other hazards

- Heavy drinkers are six times more likely to commit suicide than light drinkers or non-drinkers.
- Heavy drinkers are three times more likely to die in a car crash.

EVEN LIGHT OR MODERATE DRINKING CAN LEAD TO PROBLEMS

Work

Your ability to carry out your job may be affected by alcohol; you may have an accident at work; you may be late for work often or miss it completely because of hangovers.

Money

Alcohol is expensive. As a nation we spend more on it than clothes or cars, hospitals or schools. You may spend more on it than either you or your family can really afford.

Social life

People for whom drinking has become their social life tend to lose friends. They certainly exclude other things from their lives which are more interesting than just drinking for its own sake.

Family

Alcohol plays a large part in many family arguments and marriage breakups, and also in a great deal of domestic violence. Even on a less serious level, drinking may cause you to neglect your spouse and not give your children the attention you should.

The law

Alcohol can make otherwise reasonable people act in ways which get them into trouble with the police. And of course drinking and driving makes you not only liable to be disqualified from driving but also causes you to take huge risks with your own life and the lives of other, innocent people. There's no way of being sure when you've been drinking that you're under the legal limit. How much you can drink varies from person to person and some people might reach their limit after only about three units. Remember your driving ability will be affected by just one or two drinks. It takes the body (via the liver) about one hour to get rid of one unit of alcohol, so if you have a lot to drink at night you may still be over the legal limit the next morning.

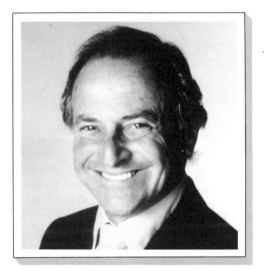

DAVID JACOBS

Let me not be pious about this because I am very fond of whisky and I look forward to my first drink of the day which I have at about 7 o'clock in the evening. A single isn't worth having though it's better than nothing but, if I'm honest, my first whisky leads on to my second. Then I stop, not because I know my limitations, it's frankly all I want. Of course, there are people who find that they lose their limitation-perception the more they have and that is one of the great problems we must face.

HOW TO START DRINKING SAFELY

■ There are many reasons, as we've seen, for wanting to drink safely while still enjoying alcohol. Start thinking of your own personal reasons for wanting to cut down your drinking. Write down as many as you can.

My husband/wife wants me to cut down.
I want to save some money – I waste so much on drink.
I want to lose weight. (Alcohol is often a big contribution to people being overweight, see p. 23.)
I feel ashamed because of my drinking.
My work is suffering.
I want to have more time to do other things.

- Make a contract with yourself or with a friend. Promise yourself that you will cut down by a certain amount and specify the timescale in which you will do it. Better still, promise yourself that from now on you will only drink up to the safe limit each week.
- Think of a reward you could give yourself when you achieve your goal (see pp. 22 and 67 for more ideas on this: the principle is exactly the same).
- Start keeping a 'drinking diary' containing a little more detail than the drinking chart used earlier to discover the number of units a week you are drinking (see pp. 86–7). This will give you a much clearer idea of your pattern of drinking and the situations where you drink more than you would like. Try to keep this drinking diary for the next two weeks at least. Put an entry in for each drinking session – lunchtime, early evening and late evening perhaps. Try to fill the diary in each day and then go through your diary and ask yourself:

> Are there particular times when I drink heavily? Like a Friday night for example?
> Are there particular places, a particular pub perhaps, where I always drink heavily?
> Are there particular people in whose company I always drink heavily?
> Do I drink because of pressure from friends?

Work out how you are going to avoid these situations – like going for a meal rather than to the pub; going to the cinema; arranging to meet friends with whom you don't drink heavily.

Then, look at how you were feeling and why you drank. Be wary if you are drinking for these sorts of reasons:

> Do I drink because I had to be polite?
> Do I drink because I need to relax?
> Do I drink to forget my worries?
> Do I drink when I feel angry?
> Do I drink because I feel bored?

If you're drinking for these reasons, then you may find that your consumption of alcohol increases and increases. Talk to someone about your problems, your husband or wife or a friend or your family doctor. Start thinking of other ways to relax if you do feel tense (see Chapter 8).

DRINKING DIARY

Day	When	Where	With whom	What
Friday	Lunchtime After work Evening	In pub In pub In pub	Terry+Brian Terry+Brian Bob+Chris	2 pints beer 2 pints beer 6 pints beer
Saturday	Lunchtime Evening	In pub In restaurant	Tony My wife	1 pint beer 1 G+T, 4 wine
Sunday	Before lunch With lunch Evening	In pub At home In pub	Bob+Chris My wife Bob+Chris	2 pints beer 3 red wine 4 pints beer
Monday	After work Evening	In pub In pub	Terry+John Bob+Chris	2 pints beer 3 pints beer
Tuesday	Lunchtime After work Evening	In restaurant In pub At home	Clients Brian+John My wife	2G+T, 2 wine 2 pints beer 3 red wine
Wednesday	Evening	At home	My wife	2 red wine
Thursday	Lunchtime Evening	In restaurant At home	Clients My wife	3 white wine 3 red wine

Cutting down

After you've analysed your diary, make a series of drinking rules for
yourself that will help you to avoid the problem situations.
Although your rules will be personal to you one of them should be
never to drink before driving or operating machinery. The list may
look something like this:

Units	Money spent on drink (approx)	Why did I drink?	How was I feeling?	Total units
2 2 6	£3 £0 £10	To be sociable End of the week Habit	Happy Happy So so	10
— 2 5	— £2 £10	—— Habit To enjoy myself	—— So so Happy	7
4 3 8	£2 £3 £4	Habit Habit To be sociable	So so Relaxed Happy	15
— 4 6	— £0 £4	—— To relax To be sociable	—— Uptight So so	10
3 4 3	£10 £0 £3	Everyone else did To unwind Habit	Tense Uptight So so	10
— — 2	— — £3	—— —— Habit	—— —— Happy	2
3 — 3	£5 £3	To be sociable Habit	So so So so	6

Total money £62 Total units 60

I won't drink at lunchtimes.
I won't drink before 7 o'clock in the evening.
I won't drink if I'm not also eating.
I won't drink on Mondays, Tuesdays and Thursdays.
I won't drink for more than three hours at a time.

When you're actually going out drinking there are several things you can do to try to ensure that you don't drink more than you want to:

- Always plan in advance how much you will drink and stick to it.
- Take smaller, less frequent sips and put your glass down between drinks. Aim to drink as slowly as possible.
- Concentrate on the drink as you sip it. Really notice the taste: don't just gulp it without noticing it.
- Try to do something else as well as drinking, like eating, talking and playing games such as dominoes or darts.
- Always dilute your drink if you can. Top up spirits with plenty of mixers and, again, drink slowly.
- There are several techniques if you're in a group where people are buying rounds:

    Explain that you're actually cutting down and you'd rather just buy your own drinks.
    Buy one round – so you don't look mean and then buy your own drinks.
    Don't buy yourself a drink when you're buying a round for everyone else. Have a rest, or have a non-alcoholic drink.

- Try a non-alcoholic drink. Perrier with ice and lemon is now very chic! Many bars now offer a wide range of non-alcoholic cocktails. Experiment.
- Try low-alcohol and alcohol-free alternatives to what you normally drink. There are now low-alcohol and alcohol-free lagers, beers, ciders and wines.

What if you can't cut down

Remember, this whole chapter is not about alcoholism and alcoholics – people who are physically dependent on drink. But it's not only alcoholics who need specialist help. If you've tried to cut down but can't, please don't abandon the attempt. There are many people who are waiting to help you. For a list of addresses and telephone numbers see pp. 140–1.

6 HOW TO AVOID HEART DISEASE

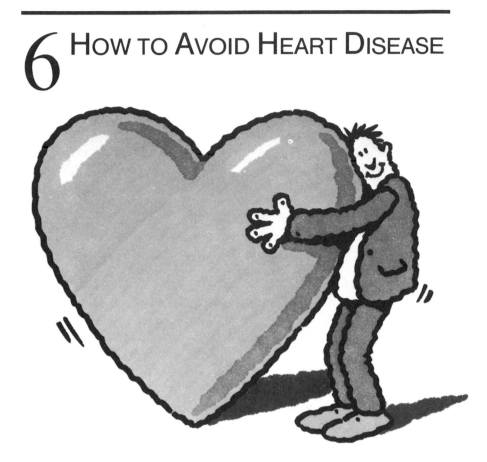

There's good news and bad news about heart disease.

THE BAD NEWS

Heart attacks are the main cause of death in this country (more than all cancers put together). What is more, they are by far the main cause of *premature* death (more than 30 times the number of those killed in road accidents). It's often said that, as we have to die of something, a heart attack is a good way to go. It's over very quickly. Well, a heart attack may be a good way to go in your eighties, but increasingly it's been people in their forties and fifties who are dying of heart disease. One man in five in this country will have a heart attack before the age of 65 and for half of them it will be fatal.

Two hundred thousand people a year in the UK die of heart disease: more than one person every three minutes. The toll is equivalent to a fully-laden jumbo jet crashing every weekday and two of them crashing every Saturday and Sunday. Heart attacks have come to seem a normal, natural way to die.

THE GOOD NEWS

Heart attacks are a twentieth-century epidemic and have increased a hundredfold over the last 50 years. So, although heart disease has come to be seen as normal, it is certainly not inevitable. We are all at risk from a heart attack, but we can all do things to cut that risk to the absolute minimum. There's overwhelming evidence now available which shows that it's the way we live which causes this high risk of a heart attack.

Britain is at the top of the world heart disease deaths' table. Other countries have cut their rates of heart attack dramatically over the last 15 years – by a third or more in the United States, Australia and New Zealand. We could do the same and, if we enjoyed that level of success, we could save 70,000 lives a year. One of them could be yours.

HOW TO GAMBLE ON YOUR HEART

Most of us don't think we live dangerously: we don't go scuba diving or abseiling. Yet so many of us do things every day which are far more dangerous – and the combination of these can be a deadly cocktail which makes a heart attack very likely.

There's a whole range of risk factors which add to the likelihood of a heart attack. Some of these we can't do a thing about, but the others – which for most people are the decisive ones – we can influence greatly. Now no one can predict with absolute certainty who will or won't get a heart attack – but it is possible to predict who is *likely* to get one. The vast majority of us have the choice: are we a near 'cert' for a heart attack or a rank outsider?

THE RISKS OF HEART DISEASE WE CAN'T DO ANYTHING ABOUT

We can't alter the following factors which increase the likelihood of heart disease:

Age

The furring up of the tiny arteries supplying our heart with blood is the underlying foundation for heart disease. In Britain the evidence shows that it begins in childhood and increases throughout life. So the risk of a heart attack becomes greater with each passing year.

Invariably, the people who get heart attacks have accelerated the furring-up process by the way they have lived their lives. This is shown by the fact that the heart attack risk for a man aged 40 *now* is the same as the risk was for a man aged 60 in the *1930s*.

Sex

A man in his late forties is five times more likely than a woman of the same age to have a heart attack.

The reasons why are not fully known but it seems that female hormones help to protect women from heart disease until they reach the menopause. Then women start to catch men up and their risk of a heart attack becomes almost the same.

Heart disease in women has been increasing, though, and in the last 20 years, there has been a rise in heart attacks in women in their thirties and forties. So women can influence their risk of a heart attack as much as men can by their lifestyle.

Family History

Heart disease often seems to run in families. It's true that if one of your parents or a brother or sister has or had a heart attack (especially at an early age) then you are more likely to have one yourself. But this is not a certainty: you don't inherit heart disease from your parents like brown eyes or blond hair. What we may inherit is a susceptibility to the other risk factors – the ones we can influence – and so it's all the more important to reduce these to the minimum.

Diabetes

Having diabetes does accelerate the furring-up process of our heart's blood supply. Men and women with diabetes are more at risk of a heart attack, particularly those who need insulin injections. But there's evidence that when the diabetes is well controlled, the risk is reduced. If you do have diabetes, it's again all the more vital that you cut down on every other possible risk.

THE RISKS OF HEART DISEASE WHICH CAN PARTLY BE CONTROLLED

Oral contraceptives or the 'Pill'

This is an effective and acceptable method of contraception for many women and the risks associated with taking the Pill are very small.

However, women who do take the Pill are at an increased risk of heart attack. For most younger women, this increased risk is so very tiny that it's insignificant: heart attacks are so rare in young women anyway and it's likely that the risk is lower now than it used to be when the Pill contained higher doses of hormones. For women over 35 who are on the Pill and who *smoke* the increased risk does become significant. This is why every woman on the Pill should definitely stop smoking.

As you get older the risks from taking oral contraceptives increase and, once you've completed your family, you should discuss alternative methods of contraception with your doctor.

All women taking the Pill should have their blood pressure taken regularly – at least once a year, if not every six months. High blood pressure and the use of the Pill combine to bring a significant risk of a heart attack or a stroke.

Soft drinking water

Statistically, there is evidence that heart disease is more common in those areas of the UK where the drinking water is soft. However, the link is still not proven and, even if it were established, it is a very minor risk compared with the things that are directly under our own control. It's wise, though, to avoid drinking artificially softened water.

THE RISKS OF HEART DISEASE WE CAN DO A GREAT DEAL ABOUT

Smoking

Remember that smoking 20 cigarettes a day trebles the risk of a heart attack (see p. 59). If you are a smoker, stopping smoking should be your number one priority. You can dramatically alter the odds in your favour. Follow the 14-day stop smoking plan in Chapter 4.

High blood cholesterol

Virtually everyone in Britain has too high a level of cholesterol in their blood and it's this excess cholesterol which causes the arteries of our heart to fur up.

What we eat greatly influences the level of cholesterol in our blood: a diet high in saturated fats can push it up to dangerous levels. Chapter 1 tells you how to follow a healthy diet which will reduce your blood cholesterol to the very minimum that you personally can get it down to. Remember, too, that you can easily get your blood cholesterol level measured through your GP.

High blood pressure

Raised blood pressure greatly contributes to the risk of a heart attack. We can do something about this ourselves, and ensure our doctor does something too (see Chapter 7).

Obesity

Being overweight increases our risk of heart disease. This is another good reason to lose weight: Chapter 2 tells you how and gives you our 14-day weight-loss plan.

Lack of exercise

Taking regular exercise cuts your risk of heart disease. See Chapter 3 for what you can do to start exercising now.

Stress and personality

As Chapter 8 points out, this is more difficult to define. But there *are* ways you can learn to relax as explained in that chapter and there's a good chance that by doing so you will cut the risk of heart disease.

Controlling the odds

The three key risk factors are smoking, high blood pressure and high blood cholesterol. Even moderate levels of each increase the risk of a heart attack by two or three times. If you are running two or three of these risks, then the overall odds begin to increase even more dramatically as the risk factors interact with each other. So, having two of these key risk factors could increase your risk *four times*; having three of them could increase it *eight times*.

You really can have a great influence in deciding your own odds of a heart attack. The changes you need to make are not beyond you and they really are worth making. Too many people in this country are dying in their forties and fifties of a heart attack for you not to do all you can to reduce your own risk.

7 Avoiding High Blood Pressure and Strokes

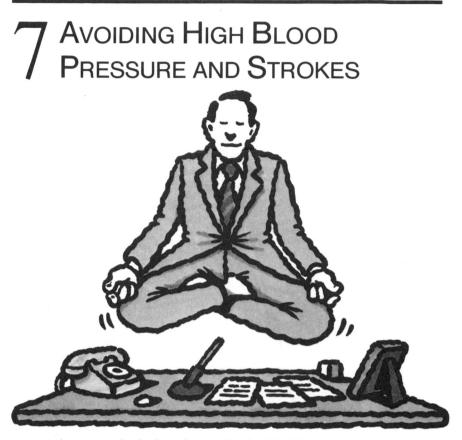

As we saw in the last chapter, having high blood pressure is one of the main contributors to the risk of heart attacks. It's also especially influential in the chance of getting a stroke. In a country such as the United States, where for many years high blood pressure has been detected and treated, strokes are now rare. This risk that high blood pressure brings is exacerbated by smoking and by having a high blood cholesterol level.

It's very important to know whether or not we have raised blood pressure, but so many of us have never had our blood pressure measured and many more haven't had it measured in the last few years.

Doctors have a range of drugs they can use to reduce high blood pressure, but there's also a great deal we can do ourselves to keep our blood pressure normal or to reduce it if it is high.

WHAT IS BLOOD PRESSURE?

Our blood pressure is the pressure exerted by our heart and arteries to push blood around our body.

A good analogy is a hose-pipe. To increase the water pressure you can increase the flow from the tap (the equivalent of making the heart work harder); or reduce the diameter of the hose-pipe by partly covering the end with the thumb (this is the equivalent of constricting the blood vessels). The water pressure is the sum of these two – the water flow and the resistance it meets – and blood pressure is the sum of the blood flow from the heart and the resistance it meets from the arteries.

If blood pressure increases it puts a strain on the heart and also causes wear and tear on the walls of the arteries. It damages their lining and makes them more likely to fur up, increasing the risk of heart attacks and strokes.

WHEN DOES BLOOD PRESSURE GO UP?

Our blood pressure does go up and down throughout the day. Everyone's blood pressure rises when they're excited, angry or afraid. This is a normal reaction and occurs as adrenalin and other hormones are released. These increase blood pressure and cause more blood to flow to the muscles and the brain. When we calm down or the danger passes, then our blood pressure goes down again.

This variation is quite normal. High blood pressure is diagnosed when our resting blood pressure is raised: that is, it's high when we're resting, sitting, reading, listening to the radio or sleeping. This is abnormal. We can't feel anything when our blood pressure is high and it only very rarely causes any symptoms. The only way to know is to get it measured.

The medical term for high blood pressure is hypertension. It's an unfortunate word because it seems to imply high blood pressure means a high level of tension. In fact, striving, competitive, impatient people may be more likely to develop high blood pressure which becomes a threat to their health but also, the most placid people may have high blood pressure.

Even doctors in Britain have got used to the idea that people's blood pressure rises with age and this has come to be accepted as normal: *it isn't*. It's true that it's par for the course for us in Britain, but there are many societies where it doesn't occur. There's convincing, and increasing, evidence that it's our lifestyle that is responsible for dangerously increasing average blood pressure in this country.

WHAT SHOULD WE DO?

The first thing to do is find out what your blood pressure is: ask a nurse or doctor to measure it. The best GPs are checking blood pressure now as a matter of routine when middle-aged people consult them about something else. In some practices one of the nurses may give regular blood pressure checks too. There's no excuse not to do this, as it is quick to do, completely safe and cheap. Also, high blood pressure and the diseases it can help to cause can be prevented. So ask your doctor to take your blood pressure next time you visit the surgery.

The Royal College of General Practitioners recommends that everyone between the ages of 20 and 65 should have their blood pressure taken at least once every five years. (American doctors recommend every two years.) If there are special circumstances, such as women taking the contraceptive pill, your doctor may want to measure your blood pressure more frequently than this.

High blood pressure shouldn't be diagnosed on one reading; at least three readings over a few weeks should be consistently high before high blood pressure is diagnosed.

If your blood pressure is high your doctor may decide to give you tablets. If he or she does prescribe them, do take them. Alternatively, he may suggest a range of things you can do yourself to get your blood pressure down to normal. Your doctor is more likely to do this if your blood pressure is only slightly raised.

WHAT CAN YOU DO YOURSELF?

There are quite a few things you can do yourself to bring your blood pressure down if it is raised. And, if your blood pressure is normal, doing these things will help to ensure that it stays that way.

- Stop smoking. Smoking increases your blood pressure and increases your risk of a heart attack or a stroke (see Chapter 4).
- Get your weight down into the ideal weight range for your height. If you have raised blood pressure just this alone may bring it back to normal (see Chapter 2).
- Don't drink too much alcohol. Alcohol tends to increase your blood pressure (see Chapter 5).
- Start exercising. Even modest amounts of exercise help to lower your blood pressure or keep it normal (see Chapter 3).
- Cut down your fat intake. A high fat diet has been shown to have an effect in raising blood pressure (see Chapter 1).
- Cut down your salt intake (see Chapter 1). In susceptible people, the effect of eating too much salt can increase blood pressure dramatically.
- Learn how to manage stress in your life and how to relax (see Chapter 8).

Even slightly raised blood pressure increases the risk of strokes and heart attacks but remember there's so much you can do yourself to prevent it.

8 COPING WITH STRESS

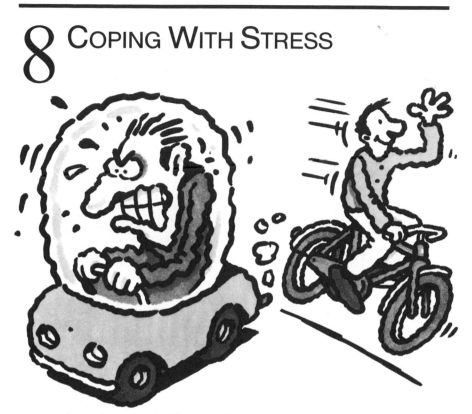

Stress is an inevitable part of our life. We know that too much of it is bad, but then so is too little: stress motivates us to do useful things. Stress is also often bound up with happy and enjoyable things – like getting married, having a baby, being promoted, even going on holiday.

One of the problems with stress is knowing what it is. Most of us might think that we know it when we feel it, but we'd be hard-pressed to define it. However, one person's stress is another person's impetus for achieving things in life. It's impossible, for example, for anyone to assess how stressful a job is unless they're the one who's doing it.

Major stress may come to us all following such things as bereavement, family illness, divorce and retirement. But the degree of stress we feel is not so much determined by outside events as by our own ability to cope with them. And we can all teach ourselves to cope better with our reactions to stress.

THE NORMAL PHYSICAL REACTION TO PHYSICAL STRESS

In common with all animals we have a natural reaction to stress. In the days when stress was caused by an attacking predator or other physical threat, the human body was prepared for a rapid retreat by the stress hormones (like adrenalin) which pump into the blood. These prepared the body for 'fight or flight': either to attack the predator or to run away.

Adrenalin increases the heart rate, pushes up the blood pressure and causes the blood vessels in the skin and the gut to contract so that more blood is available to flow to the muscles. Adrenalin and other stress hormones are responsible for giving us the feeling of 'nerves' like sweaty palms and butterflies in the tummy. These changes occur in seconds and when the physical activity for which they have prepared is over, the stress hormones disappear and the body returns to equilibrium.

REACTIONS TO EMOTIONAL STRESS

The problem is that this same reaction, the outpouring of stress hormones, occurs whenever we get angry, tense, frightened or excited. So when we drive in the rush-hour, have an argument or watch our favourite football team lose again, the level of stress hormones in our bodies goes up. We don't, in these circumstances, get rid of them by physical activity, so while we're impatiently sitting in traffic the stress hormones continue to circulate in our bloodstream.

The same reaction can also be provoked by our own thoughts and imagination. Worrying about our present or future problems can just as surely pour these stress hormones into our bloodstreams as an attacking tiger. We can become tense, frustrated, unhappy and feel that we just can't cope with life.

WHAT PROBLEMS DOES STRESS CAUSE?

The main problem that stress causes is a feeling of distress. We may feel mental anguish, a sense of being trapped and unable to concentrate at work. Or, we may get physical symptoms like tension headaches, pain, breathlessness or sleeplessness.

Common sense tells us that you can't separate mind and body

and it's often postulated that stress is implicated in a wide range of diseases. Hard evidence is scanty, but, of course, it's difficult to come by because of the inherent problems of defining stress and measuring it. Increasingly, though, it does seem that stress – particularly the sort of chronic stress caused by unemployment or family worries – does play a part in the development of heart disease and it's certainly possible that it may be one of the factors which helps to cause other diseases too.

We don't need scientific evidence to know that we'd feel better if we were able to cope with the stress in our life.

GET TO KNOW YOURSELF

Start keeping an informal 'stress diary' so that you pinpoint the circumstances where stress occurs in your life. It may not be the sort of diary that you write every day, but over a few weeks note down the times and occasions in which you felt under pressure, tense, frustrated, panicky or unable to cope. Write down:

the time of day
where you were
what you were doing
what you were thinking about
your mood before it happened
who you were with and where
how long the feelings lasted
the consequences, e.g., did you have to go home from work or have a sleepless night.

Over a few weeks, see if a pattern emerges.

- Do you always get stressed at a particular time of day?
- Do you get stressed in a particular place?
- Do you get stressed when you do a particular thing?
- Do you get stressed when you get into a certain train of thought?
- Do certain people regularly make you feel stressed?

Knowing the circumstances in which you get stressed helps enormously in self-understanding and also helps you to plan preventative action. Analyse why you react in the way you do and then think of what you can do in that situation to be less tense. For example, if you always get tense when you're in rush-hour traffic, ask yourself first of all if you can avoid the situation by setting out earlier so you've got plenty of time for the journey. If you're unexpectedly stuck in traffic and are going to be late for work or for an important meeting, engage yourself in an inner conversation. Ask yourself why you are getting fraught. Tell yourself that you may as well have 10 minutes calm rather than 10 minutes of seething anger. Think of the extra time as a bonus, a gift: listen to the radio; plan your next holiday; imagine what you'd do if you won the pools. The end result – being late – will be the same whether you are calm or angry. But you'll have coped with the situation without all those stress hormones circulating around your body.

Think of similar ways, and similar inner conversations, for all of the situations you have identified where stress is a problem. The ideal, of course, is to avoid stressful situations. But that isn't always possible, alas, this side of Paradise! The next best thing is to cope better in those situations.

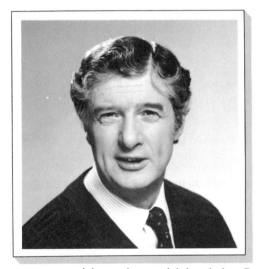

JOHN DUNN

I don't think I have a particularly stressful job, because at 7 o'clock each evening, it's over. There is no way I can take today's programme home with me. However, stress can build up during the day but only if you let it. I run each day to an unpublished timetable. *I* know what I have to have done and by what time, to be on a smooth track. Particularly in London you have to take conscious steps to eliminate stress. When calculating journey times, you have to be realistic (and then add on a few minutes) to avoid arriving at the next job in a lather. But things are going to go wrong – there are going to be crises, so expect them, perhaps anticipate them and, for heaven's sake, if possible, enjoy them!

'ACTION KILLS WORRY'

This is a favourite saying of a very good friend. It's true, though I have to admit that I often observe it in the breach.

Often we feel stressed and tense because worries seem impossible to tackle. Or, as we tackle them, other larger ones appear to take their place. We start to feel as if we're living in a nightmare. In this case worries can evaporate, or at least lose their power over us, if we write them down. The first thing that may surprise you is that there are not as many as you thought. Also, when you see them on paper, you can better answer the question 'Is this a real problem or am I blowing it up out of all proportion?' Put your problems and worries in order of importance. Is there something you can do about the first, then the second, then the third.

I'm not suggesting that all the worries in your life can be solved by ticking off a list, but you'll clearly see the ones you can do something about and eliminate. Some worries and problems may not have solutions, but never underestimate the huge difference it can make to talk to someone about your problems. Talk to your partner or to a friend or a doctor, priest or minister.

HOW TO EASE AWAY THE STRESS

The best way to cope with stress and with the feelings that it causes is by learning to relax. You can start building this into your life.

Exercise

This is one of the best ways of relieving stress and easing away that tense feeling. The sensations of well-being and relaxation brought on by exercise last for far longer than the actual time you spend exercising. Exercising, of course, is the natural way of coping with those stress hormones. Even short walks are a good way of relaxing and releasing tension, but start thinking of how you can start exercising regularly (see Chapter 3).

Deep breathing

This sounds a very simple technique but slow, deep breaths are an effective way of calming down and relieving tension.

Sit in an upright, comfortable chair and close your eyes. Breathe slowly through your nose trying to take in the air down to your toes. Then, slowly, steadily and deliberately breathe out. Continue to do this and concentrate your thoughts on breathing, in and out, in and out. As you breathe out, imagine all your tensions going out of the body with your breath. If your mind starts racing or thinking of something else bring your attention back to your breathing.

A couple of minutes of this is guaranteed to relax you. Do it regularly in situations where you feel tense and you'll soon find that you have trained your body to relax by this method, so that even a few deep breaths will make you feel calm.

Deep relaxation

This is a way of getting all your muscles to relax and to eliminate feelings of tension.

Sit comfortably in an upright chair with your feet on the floor and your hands held on your lap, palms upwards. Let your fingers relax, neither trying to straighten them nor make a fist.

Now concentrate on your toes and feet. Feel the muscles in them relax and, as they do so, feel your feet become heavier. Now feel the muscles in your calves relax and then the muscles in your thighs. As your legs relax, they'll roll outwards slightly.

Next feel the muscles in your bottom relaxing; you'll feel more comfortable as you seem to press down in the chair. Now the muscles of your back are relaxing and you feel more and more relaxed and comfortable in the chair.

Feel the fingers of your left hand relaxing and then your right hand. The wave of relaxation now goes up both your arms and into your shoulders. Let your shoulders drop. Now feel the muscles of your neck relaxing; then the muscles of your face; feel your cheeks relaxing and your mouth open very slightly. Then think of the muscles of your forehead relaxing.

Now feel your whole body relaxed and still. Concentrate on your breathing: feel the breath going in and then slowly out, taking all your tensions with it.

If your mind fills with other thoughts, concentrate on your breathing and if necessary go through again relaxing each part of your body in turn. You'll find you can do it more quickly this time.

Try to keep relaxed like this for five or ten minutes.

Relax like this whenever you're feeling tense – you can do it at home or perhaps in the office at lunchtime or even on the bus. The feeling of calm and release from tension should last with you the rest of the day. You'll find that as you practise this technique it will become easier and easier and soon you'll be able to make your whole body relax in seconds.

If you're feeling tense but think you can't find time in the day to do this sort of exercise, then you definitely need to find the time. If you can't find five minutes to switch off and re-charge, you really need to assess your priorities. (Ask yourself why you don't want to find the time – this is more likely the case.)

Meditation

You can get yourself into the right frame of mind to meditate by using the deep breathing and deep relaxation exercises above. Then you can use one of several techniques.

You could just concentrate on your breathing. Don't push other thoughts from your mind, but if other thoughts do intrude, just come back to concentrate on the rhythm – slowly in and slowly out – of your breathing. As you breathe you could repeat to yourself 'in-out'.

You could focus your mind on pleasant and soothing images like gentle waves on a seashore or leaves rustling in the wind.

You could repeat a word, or a sound, or a syllable over and over again like 'relax' or 'peace'. Many religions use similar techniques: a mantra is repeated in Buddhism and Hinduism and there's the rosary and the 'Jesus' prayer in Christianity. Again, repeat your chosen word or phrase and gently bring your mind back to it if it wanders. Relax into the steady rhythm for five or ten minutes.

Recent medical research has shown that this sort of meditation or prayer not only makes you feel more relaxed and less tense but also helps to lower your blood pressure. Patients who had slightly raised blood pressure and who were taught to practise these techniques were found to be able to reduce their blood pressure without the aid of drugs.

How Not to Cope With Stress

The great danger of feeling under stress is that it may push you into behaviour which will start to damage your health. Stress could cause you to smoke, eat more or drink more. If stress causes you to do those things, there's no doubt that it could be increasing your risk of a whole range of diseases.

- Don't smoke – see Chapter 4 for how to give up.
- Don't eat more – see Chapter 1 for healthy eating advice.
- Don't drink more – see Chapter 5 for ways of how to cut down.
- Don't abandon exercise – remember it helps you to relax (see Chapter 3).
- Don't drink endless cups of coffee (caffeine is a stimulant and increases tension).
- Don't rely on pills and tranquillisers as a permanent solution to stress. Tranquillisers can be useful for a short time if you're going through an extremely stressful period. But they're not a long-term solution to stress. Used for days or weeks, they're fine: used for months and years, they start bringing their own problems as you can become dependent on them. Ask your doctor's advice. Don't be afraid to take them if you need them for a short time but, if you think you're using too many or you're worried you're taking them for too long, tell your doctor you want to stop and wean yourself off them.

9 WOMEN'S HEALTH

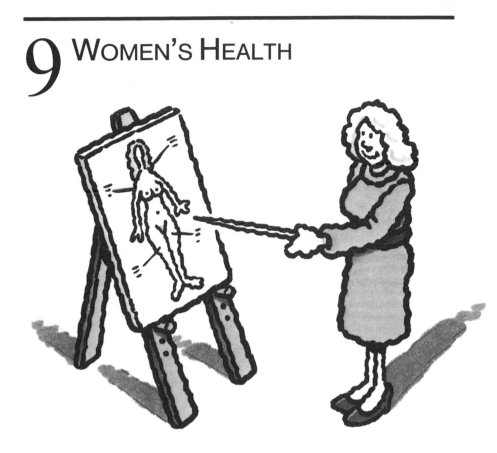

Women tend to be more interested in and knowledgeable about health than men. Generally, women are more aware that we are frail flesh and blood. Men, however, often try not to think about the body, health and disease – until it's too late. Women are more in touch with their own bodies – they have no choice!

There's a great deal women can do for themselves to deal with the problems and prevent the illnesses which are unique to women.

WOMEN AND HEALTHY LIFESTYLES

Women can not only help themselves but also do a great deal about the illnesses that affect us all. It's just as well that women tend to be more interested in health than men, because invariably it's the women who decide whether the family's lifestyle is healthy.

Diet

Women usually decide a family's eating pattern – whether it's healthy or unhealthy. It's a big responsibility because it's becoming increasingly clear how many diseases are influenced by the food we eat. What we eat in childhood can greatly affect our health later on in life.

Smoking

Children of smokers tend to have more chest infections, for example, than those of non-smokers. Also, what sort of example are you setting your children if you smoke? Children of smokers are more likely to start smoking themselves. This is a responsibility for fathers too, of course! Make sure you set a healthy example. (See Chapter 4 for how to stop smoking.)

Drinking sensibly

Women have to be more careful than men about the amount of alcohol they drink (see p. 80). Women who are pregnant, or who want to get pregnant, need to be especially careful to drink the minimum amount possible (for the reasons given on pp. 82–3). Again, you're setting your children an example here as well.

Exercise

Do find time to fit regular exercise into your lifestyle. Remember it will help you to cope with a busy life, as well as bringing you so many healthy benefits (see Chapter 3). Do your children think it's normal to take some exercise or do they think that the only way to relax is to lie in front of the television?

Stress

Stress affects many women who often have to cope simultaneously with so many conflicting demands: a job; running a home; a husband; children; and their own feelings. Take time out to relax: you're not being selfish. You deserve it and you can only give if you're not feeling tense and stressful. (See Chapter 8.)

Premenstrual Tension (PMT) and the Premenstrual Syndrome (PMS)

One of the reasons an average woman is so much more in touch with her own body than an average man is because of the powerful control exerted on her body by the ebb and flow of her hormones.

Most women notice some changes in mood, or physical changes, in the two weeks leading up to menstruation, the monthly period. These are mostly quite small and they don't disrupt her life to any very great degree. But in about 35 per cent of women (some would say up to 50 per cent), the changes that happen just before the monthly period are distressing and *do* disrupt normal life. These are the women who suffer from premenstrual tension, or the premenstrual syndrome. (A syndrome just means a collection of associated symptoms.)

The changes start between 12 and 15 days before menstruation begins and are gone within two days of menstruation starting. The symptoms vary both in what they are and in severity. They obviously vary between different women, but they can also vary in the same woman from one monthly cycle to another. They do follow the same pattern though, of coming before the period starts and of disappearing for a time between periods.

Emotional symptoms

irritability
anxiety
feeling tense
crying for no reason
mood swings
feeling listless or exhausted
forgetfulness
confusion.

Physical symptoms

severe breast swelling or pain
feeling of weight gain
swelling of the ankles, feet or hands
feeling the tummy bloated
headaches
backache
feeling sick.

In the diagnosis of PMS it's not so much the individual symptoms which are significant, but how they come and go regularly within the monthly cycle.

It's thought that PMS is more common in women between the age of 30 and 45. It's often precipitated by childbirth or a very significant life-event like the death of a close relative.

It's not been proved what causes PMS, though there are many theories. It's been postulated that it's a hormonal imbalance, or that the chemicals which transmit messages in the brain are to blame. Because it's not known what causes it, there is no one drug that is used to treat it, though there are several different types of drugs which are used. Some are successful in treating it for some women, and others for other women.

It's helpful to keep a note of your symptoms for several menstrual cycles at least. List your three worst emotional symptoms and the three worst physical ones. Put them in order of severity. Do this each month. This helps you to assess what the problems are, and it also helps your doctor to assess them too.

Some doctors are more sympathetic than others to women suffering from PMS. Some enlightened practices now run Well Woman Clinics where such problems are tackled very professionally. If you do find your doctor isn't sympathetic, do think about seeing another doctor in the practice, or even changing doctors. Remember, though, that your doctor may question you about other things because the symptoms you have may be connected with other health problems or problems in your life.

The medications used by doctors to treat PMS include:

pyridoxine or vitamin B6
diuretics or 'water tablets' especially spironolactone
progesterone
bromocriptine
mefanamic acid, or another non-steroid anti-inflammatory drug.

You can do something yourself to relieve the symptoms. First of all, identifying and clarifying them and just writing them down helps. Discuss them with your husband and perhaps your children. Ask for understanding and tolerance when you are experiencing the symptoms. Discussing your problems with a close female friend will help too. Learn how to relax (see Chapter 8). Use one of the relaxation techniques mentioned there on the days you are feeling tense and irritable. Don't forget the value of exercise in helping to relax.

CERVICAL CANCER

Cancer of the cervix (the neck of the womb) kills 2,000 women a year in Britain. Yet it is a curable disease – over 80 per cent of those who are treated while the disease is at an early stage are completely cured. Only a few are cured if the disease is at an advanced stage when it is discovered.

What causes it?

Cervical cancer is connected in some way with sexual intercourse – it is very rare in virgins. The earlier a woman starts her sex life and the more partners she has had, the greater the risk of developing cancer of the cervix. However, any woman, if she has or has had a sex life at all, is at risk.

The risk is much lower in women who use a contraceptive cap (the 'Dutch cap') or whose partner wears a condom during intercourse. In addition, the condom also offers some protection against sexually-transmitted diseases and AIDS. Make a point of discussing methods of contraception with your doctor or at your local family planning clinic.

What you can do

Stop smoking

Smoking doubles the risk of developing cancer of the cervix. It's another good reason to stop (see Chapter 4).

Have a cervical smear test

It's very important for all women who are sexually active (or have been at any time in the past) to have a cervical smear test. You should have one every three to five years for the rest of your life. If you are aged between 20 and 64, you should be invited to have a cervical smear test as part of the nationwide screening programme.

You'll then continue to get an invitation to have one every five years. Otherwise, your own doctor will be happy to arrange for you to have one.

The cervical smear test is very simple, quick and painless. The doctor takes a sample of the moisture from the neck of the womb and smears it on to a slide for inspection under a microscope.

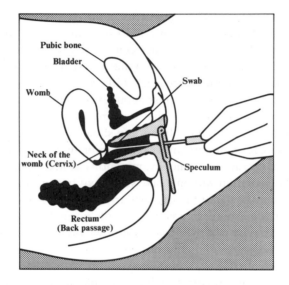

The purpose of the test is to look at the cells from the cervix which are contained in the smear and check whether or not they are normal. What is being looked for is a *pre-cancerous* condition. It is possible to determine if there are abnormal cells present which are likely to develop into cancer in future years. This is why it's so important to have the test. (In addition, the test can also pick up minor infections which can then be easily treated.)

In about six or seven women out of every thousand who have the test the smear is positive (showing abnormal cells). If that happens or if, as is sometimes the case, the result is not clear you will be asked to have another test.

If abnormal cells are found, they can be treated easily and painlessly without a long hospital stay and without any after-effects. In particular, the treatment makes no difference to the ability to have children.

BREAST CANCER

Breast cancer is the most common cancer to occur in women. The earlier it is detected, the easier the treatment and the greater the chance of a complete cure.

Breast self-examination

All women worry about breast cancer. Breast self-examination is something positive you can do yourself to detect any abnormalities in the breast. If you do detect a lump which turns out to be cancer, there will be a good chance that you've detected it at an early stage when a complete cure is most likely.

The first thing to stress about examining your own breasts is that nine out of ten lumps that women find in this way are not cancer. But, if you do find a lump, you should go to your doctor straight away for a professional examination and assessment and for reassurance or further examinations as necessary. Breast self-examination will only take you about five minutes each month. By examining your breasts regularly you'll get to know what is normal for you. Many women have – quite normally – breasts which feel lumpy. By getting to know your own breasts, you'll be able to detect any changes to the normal feel of them.

The best time to examine your breasts is just after your period (they can sometimes be lumpy or, of course, tender just before a period). You need to remember to examine them every month. If your periods have stopped, choose a regular day – perhaps the first day or the last day of the month – to help you remember. There are two stages to examining your breasts – looking and feeling.

Looking

Undress to the waist and then stand or sit in front of a mirror in good light. Remember you're looking for any changes in your breasts from the previous month. If this is the first time that you've looked at your breasts closely remember that no two breasts in the world are exactly alike – not even your two! One will probably be larger than the other and one will hang a little lower.

1

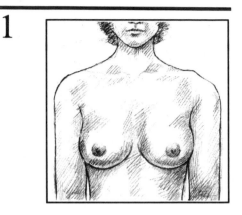

■ Look at your breasts in the mirror as your arms hang loosely to your sides. Go through this **checklist:**

Is the outline of the breasts normal? Is there any change in the size or shape or colour?

Are there any changes in the nipples? Is there any bleeding or discharge from the nipple?

Is there any unusual puckering or dimpling on the breast or nipple?

Are there any veins standing out in a way that's not usual for you?

2 ■ Now raise your arms above your head. Turn from side to side to see your breasts from different angles. Go through the **checklist** again.

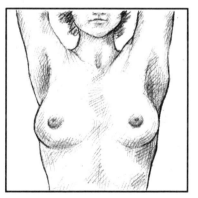

3

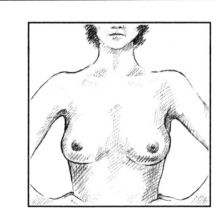

■ Put your hands on your hips and press. Go through the **checklist** again.

4

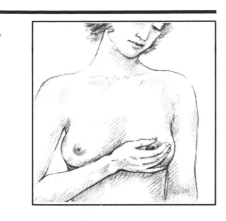

- Squeeze each nipple gently to see if there's any bleeding or discharge.

5

- Now lie down on your bed with your head on a pillow. Put a folded towel under the shoulder blade of the side you are examining – this helps to flatten the breast tissue and make it easier to examine.
- Use your left hand to examine your right breast and vice versa. Put the hand you're not using on the pillow under your head.
- As you examine your breast, keep the fingers of the hand together. Use the flat of the fingers, not the tips.

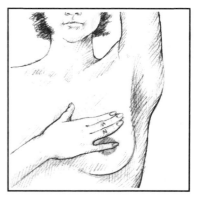

6

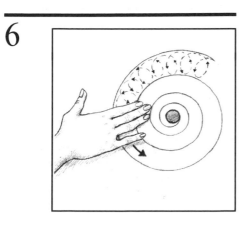

- With your fingers, trace a continuous spiral around the breast moving your fingers in small circles and using firm pressure. Start by feeling around the nipple and then work outwards in the spiral until you have felt every part of your breast. A ridge of firm tissue in a half-moon shape under the breast is quite normal: this helps to support your breast.

7

- Now bring the arm resting on the pillow down and feel the part of your breast that goes up as far as the collarbone. Then feel the part that goes into the armpit. With the flat of the fingers again, feel for any lumps. Feel right up into the hollow of the armpit and work your way back towards your breast.
- Now change sides and examine the other breast in exactly the same way with your other hand.
- If you do find something unusual in one breast, always check the other breast for the same thing – it may be just the way your breasts are made.

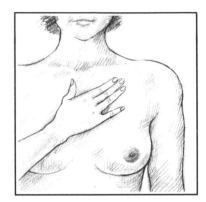

Always see your doctor as soon as possible if you do find something unusual. Don't worry if you're uncertain: it's better to have your mind put at rest and you'll be sure you're not neglecting something serious. Remember though that nine out of ten lumps are not cancerous – but if it is cancer, the sooner you get treatment, the more likely it is that you will be cured.

Mammography

The NHS is setting up breast cancer screening clinics where every woman between the age of 50 and 64 will be offered an X-ray examination, or mammography, every three years.

It's very important for women in this age group to be screened in this way and it's hoped that it will save many lives. So, accept your invitation when you get one. Like any other X-ray it is, of course, completely painless and very quick.

Women over 65 are not being invited automatically, but it's wise for them to ask their doctor or the breast-screening clinic for an appointment too.

THE MENOPAUSE

The menopause, or the change of life, is another time when women have no choice but to be in touch with their bodies.

It means the end of the monthly periods; no more eggs are released by the ovaries and the woman can no longer have children. Unfortunately, it's not quite as simple as that and the 'change' doesn't happen overnight or even over several months, but usually takes several years. The average age for the menopause is 50, but it can happen anywhere between the ages of 45 and 54. Although it can happen outside these ages, this is rare. Always wait at least one year without periods if you're over 50, or two years if you're under, before you stop using birth control methods. Before you stop using contraception, ask your doctor for advice.

About 20 per cent of women are lucky and don't notice any problems at all around the menopause; the other 80 per cent do get some symptoms, varying in degrees of severity. There are many possible symptoms caused by the menopause. You're very unlikely to get all of them but you may get several, perhaps spread over a period of years.

Periods and abnormal bleeding

Some women's periods just stop; others have more and more irregular periods until they finally stop; yet others have periods which fluctuate and are light one month and heavy the next.

It's therefore difficult to say what is abnormal bleeding, but you should see your doctor if you have any of the following:

- bleeding or spotting between periods
- bleeding or spotting after sexual intercourse
- bleeding more than a year after your last period
- frequent periods with only days between them
- very heavy bleeding or 'flooding', particularly if it contains blood clots.

Hot flushes and night sweats

Most women have one or both of these symptoms as they are going through the change. They can be upsetting, but they are not harmful. There are some things you can do yourself to help.

- Try stopping alcohol, tea, coffee and spicy foods in turn to see if they are making the hot flushes worse. They often do so and, if so, you should try avoiding them for a while.
- Wear several layers of light clothing so that you can take them off as you feel hot.
- If you have night sweats try sleeping on a large towel so you don't have to change the sheets. Use cotton sheets and nightclothes.
- Learn to relax (see Chapter 8). Feeling tense makes things worse.
- Ask your doctor for help if they really are a problem.

Dryness of the vagina

This is often a problem during the menopause. As the levels of hormones drop, so the natural lubrication of the vagina decreases and sex can be uncomfortable. Try using a lubricating jelly, like KY (available easily at any chemist). If your vagina is sore as well as dry your doctor may prescribe an oestrogen (hormone) cream.

The menopause certainly doesn't mean the end of an enjoyable sex life. In fact, for some women enjoyment of sex increases after the menopause when the worry of an unexpected or unwelcome pregnancy has disappeared.

Osteoporosis or brittle bones

Both men and women tend to lose calcium from their bones as they get older. In some women (not all) this process speeds up after the menopause. However, the effects of this may not show up until you are older – in your seventies perhaps. Only 20–30 per cent of older women do have signs of osteoporosis but this means they may develop a hunched back and their bones can break easily, even after the slightest fall.

Osteoporosis can be made worse by smoking and heavy drinking but you can help to prevent it by taking regular exercise and making sure you have a healthy and varied diet.

Emotional symptoms

The menopause is a time when women may experience feelings of:

- tension and anxiety
- depression
- mood swings, from feeling really happy one minute to utterly miserable the next.

Tension, anxiety and feeling low are not symptoms of the menopause as such. It's true that middle-aged women do often suffer from these things – but then so do middle-aged men! Don't put these symptoms down to 'the change' without first thinking carefully if there are other reasons in your life for them. Do you have so much to do you can't cope? Do you find it difficult to relax? At any age, the ways of coping with stress are the same (see Chapter 8).

Hormone replacement therapy (HRT)

Most of the symptoms of the menopause are caused by the fall in the level of the female sex hormone (oestrogen) in the blood.

The idea of hormone replacement therapy is to top up the body's level of oestrogen, so that it's kept at a constant level. Oestrogen can be given as tablets – similar tablets to the contraceptive pill but in a lower dose which doesn't act as a contraceptive. It can also be given as a slow-release implant under the skin or as a cream absorbed through the vagina. Nowadays, another natural hormone, progesterone, is usually combined with a lower dose of oestrogen to make the treatment safer and this causes monthly bleeding like a normal period.

Hormone replacement therapy usually lasts for at least six months and perhaps for several years. Usually, after it's stopped, the symptoms don't return. It's normally given when the physical symptoms of the menopause are very severe and it can help greatly. It has been argued by some that all women should receive HRT at the menopause: indeed in the USA, some women insist on taking HRT for life as they feel it's a 'keep-young' pill. It isn't, and there are serious reasons for not giving HRT indiscriminately to all women for ever.

Here are the pros and cons of HRT:

Pros

- It reduces hot flushes and sweating.
- It prevents vaginal dryness.
- It reduces the risk of osteoporosis or brittle bones.
- Some women say they feel much better when they're receiving it.

Cons

- You have to continue to have monthly bleeds.
- You need regular health checks.
- You may become psychologically dependent on it.
- There's an increased risk of cancer of the uterus (or body of the womb) if progesterone is not added as a safeguard.
- There's a slightly increased risk of gallbladder disease.
- Any long-term risks are not yet known.

What the menopause doesn't do

All the potential problems of the menopause make it sound as if you've got just one long miserable period ahead of you. But it doesn't have to be like that. It's important to know that, for many women, the menopause and the period after that can be the calmest and happiest period in life. Remember the following positive points about the 'change':

- It doesn't make you fat. Many women do put on weight at this age (but there again so do many men) and it isn't the menopause that's to blame. You can do something about being overweight at any age (see Chapter 2).
- It doesn't mean the end of your sex life.
- It's the 'change of life' not the 'end of life': many women have their happiest and most fulfilled time after the menopause.

10 HOW TO CUT THE RISK OF CANCER

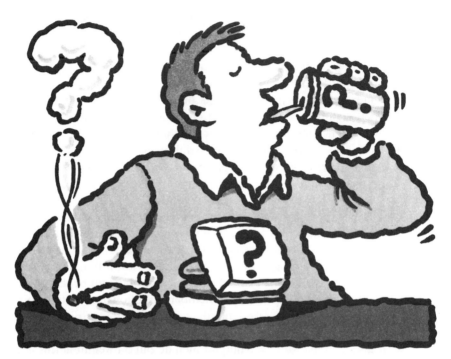

Cancer is the second commonest cause of death in this country after heart disease. Cancer is responsible for one in four of all deaths. It is not a single disease but rather a range of diseases with different causes, different preventative measures, different treatments and different success rates in curing it.

Some cancers are still very difficult to cure. Others can often be cured, especially if detected early. Others are nearly always curable.

'Prevention is better than cure' is most certainly true in the case of cancer. Not all cancers are preventable of course (or rather we don't have the knowledge yet to know how to prevent them). However, you can do several things yourself to reduce your risk of developing certain types, including some of the most common ones.

WHAT IS CANCER?

Cancer occurs when a group of the body's own cells start to act abnormally and to grow in an uncontrolled way.

We all began as a single unique cell, formed when our mother's egg (or ovum) was fertilised by our father's sperm. This single cell thus formed multiplied very rapidly, soon growing into millions of cells. The core of each cell contains coded information, parts of which switch on in particular cells to tell that cell to become either a muscle cell, a skin cell, an eye cell, a heart cell or a liver cell. The code in the cell controls growth and multiplication of our tissues throughout our life.

Once formed, some cells never divide again and multiply – for example, those in our brain. Others retain the ability to divide and multiply throughout our lives – that's how a cut on our skin heals. So many cells are dividing and multiplying in our bodies all the time, repairing old tissue or growing new. This process is still under the control of that coded information in the core of the cell which tells it when to divide and when to rest.

Cancer occurs when this mechanism goes wrong. Then, a cell starts dividing and dividing, multiplying and multiplying, and the coded information in the core can't 'switch off'. This cancerous tissue grows so rapidly that it may invade surrounding tissues, and pieces of it may break off and be carried in the bloodstream to other parts of the body and start growing there. These are secondaries or metastases, and they may start interfering with the function of those other organs in which they start growing. For example, if they're in the lungs they may cause breathlessness.

WHAT CAUSES CANCER?

There are many causes of cancer and we only know some of them. The irritants which can cause cells to become cancerous are called carcinogens and there are very many of them. The most common carcinogen is cigarette smoke – in fact it contains a lethal cocktail of chemicals which cause cancer.

There are many other chemicals which have been shown to cause cancer in humans and far, far more which have been shown to cause cancer in animals. Often they have been exposed to chemicals in far larger amounts than a human being could possibly receive so, although these studies are valuable for research purposes, they are rather hypothetical as far as human beings are concerned. It's important not to get worried about insignificant, hypothetical risks that often get blown up out of all proportion by newspapers, but it is important to be concerned with those known causes of cancer which you can do something to avoid.

As well as chemicals, viruses have been strongly implicated in a few cancers (though this certainly doesn't mean that cancer is infectious – it is not). Radiation and excessive exposure to sunlight can also cause cancer. It is also probable that there are other cancer-causing factors in the environment of which we are not yet aware.

For example, for reasons which are not yet fully clear, people in Japan are twice as likely to get cancer of the stomach than people in England and Wales. Yet women there are six times less likely to get breast cancer as women here.

It is thought by those working in cancer research that, as more and more causes of cancer become known, we will be able to take avoiding action to prevent them. In the meantime, there's a great deal that you can do *now* to cut your risk of getting cancer.

How to Avoid Cancer

There's no way to guarantee absolutely that you won't get cancer; but enough is now known to enable you to reduce considerably your risk of getting certain kinds of cancer.

A committee of cancer experts of the European Community has drawn up a ten-point plan – The European Code – for avoiding cancer. Their hope is that, if people follow these points, the number of deaths from cancer will be cut by 15 per cent at least.

Point 1: Stop smoking

- Cigarette smoking causes a third of all cancer deaths: it's by far the biggest cause of cancer that we know.
- Well over 90 per cent of lung cancer is due to smoking. Lung cancer causes 40,000 deaths a year in the UK.
- Regular smokers are up to 40 times more likely to develop lung cancer than non-smokers.

- Smoking also increases the risk of other cancers: of the mouth, the voice-box, the gullet, the liver, the bladder and the pancreas.
- The good news is that the risks begin to fall from Day 1 of stopping (see Chapter 4 for a 14-day plan on how to give up).

Point 2: Go easy on alcohol

- Drinking too much alcohol has been linked to 3 per cent of all cancer.
- If you drink heavily as well as smoke, the risk gets even higher.
- Cancer of the mouth, voice-box, gullet and liver are more common in heavy drinkers.
- You don't need to give up alcohol altogether – just drink sensibly. See Chapter 5 for the safe limits of drinking and for how to cut down if you're exceeding them.

Point 3: Avoid being overweight

- Being extremely overweight or obese increases the risk of some cancers, for example, cancer of the womb.
- Of course, if you are overweight it doesn't mean that you're necessarily going to get cancer, but it's another very good reason to lose weight (see Chapter 2 for our 14-day action weight-loss plan).

Plan 4: Cut down on fatty foods

- In Western countries, where the diet is high in fat – from meat and meat products, butter, cheese and milk, as we saw in Chapter 1 – there are high rates of cancer of the breast and of the bowel. Researchers now believe these two things are connected; in societies where the diet is much lower in fat, these cancers are rarer.
- For these reasons, as well as all the other positive reasons, cut down on the amount of fat in your diet. A full list of guidelines of how to do this is in Chapter 1.

Point 5: Eat more fibre and more fresh fruit and vegetables

- There's evidence now that fibre may actually protect against cancer of the bowel. Again, it's been shown that in communities otherwise comparable to ours, those who eat less fibre are more at risk from this cancer and those who eat more fibre are at less risk. And there are other benefits of eating more fibre. See what they are and how to increase your intake in Chapter 1.

■ There's also evidence that vitamins A and C (found in fresh fruit and vegetables such as carrots, spinach, broccoli and cabbage) may give protection against cancers. Natural foods are the best way of getting these vitamins, so eat more fresh fruit and vegetables.

■ Some people get worried about food additives like colourings, flavourings and preservatives causing cancer but there is no evidence that they do. In fact stomach cancer has become less common and it's believed that that has to do with food preservatives and refrigeration. Artificial sweeteners have caused some concern, but there's no evidence that they cause cancer in humans. Research into the whole question of additives is continuing.

Point 6: Take care in the sun

■ The sun gives off harmful ultraviolet rays and too much exposure to these can cause various types of skin cancer. These are more common in fair-haired or fair-skinned people or those who have a skin which always burns in the sun or tans slowly.

■ Skin cancers are common in fair-skinned people living in a hot climate – in Australia, for example – and they are becoming more common in this country as Spain has replaced Blackpool as the most popular holiday destination.

■ Always tan slowly by spending just short periods in the sun for the first few days of a holiday. Avoid getting sunburnt. Use sun-filter creams and lotions: these filter out the harmful ultraviolet light so use them generously and reapply them frequently. Use high protection factor sun-filters, especially if you have fair skin.

■ Ensure your children tan slowly too and don't let them get sunburnt. Their skin is sensitive and needs lots of high protection factor sun-filters.

■ Sunbeds produce similar rays to sunlight itself; they may also increase the risk of skin cancers but not enough is known about them yet.

- Most skin cancers are completely curable, especially if detected in the early stages. Always see your doctor with a spot or sore which doesn't heal within two weeks.
- One kind of skin cancer is malignant melanoma which starts as a change in the appearance of a normal skin mole. See your doctor if one of your skin moles changes in any way. In particular, if:

    it becomes itchy
    it starts to increase in size or becomes ragged around the edges
    it gets inflamed or red at the edges
    it starts bleeding, oozing or going crusty.

    You should consult your doctor if any of your skin moles are:

    bigger than the blunt end of a pencil
    a mixture of different shades of black and brown.

    These signs don't necessarily mean that the mole is becoming cancerous, but it's always wise to check. Remember, the sooner cancer is detected and treated, the better the chance of a complete cure.

Point 7: Observe the Health and Safety Regulations at work

- There are about 40 chemicals and processes which are known to cause cancer. Many of these have been banned and the others are, or should be, controlled by legislation. These include asbestos, vinyl chloride (the raw material for PVC), some chemical dyes, some compounds of arsenic, chromium and nickel and some types of tar and soot. There are so many other chemicals in use in factories and workplaces which haven't been tested that it's possible some of them could cause cancer too.
- It's very important, therefore, to observe safety regulations when working with chemicals, particularly avoiding skin contact and breathing in fumes and dust. You need to wear appropriate protective clothing and masks where necessary.
- The *Health and Safety at Work Act* requires your employer to tell you if any of the substances you are working with are toxic and to take all reasonable protective measures. If you have worries or questions

about health risks, talk to your employer, your works' doctor, your union representative or a Health and Safety Inspector. The address and phone number of the Health and Safety Executive is in your local directory.

Point 8: See your doctor if you're worried about any change in your normal health which lasts for more than two weeks

There are certain symptoms you should always consult your doctor about if they last for more than two weeks. It is unlikely that these symptoms indicate cancer – other explanations are always more likely – but it's always best to check to be on the safe side. Remember that the sooner cancer is detected, the greater the chance of a cure. So always give yourself the best odds, not the worst. See your doctor if you have the following symptoms:

■ a lump anywhere in the body
■ a sore that doesn't heal
■ a change in a skin mole – see previous page
■ any unusual bleeding, for example, in your water or your bowel motions or any blood or discharge from any orifice
■ any bleeding from the vagina or front passage after the menopause or change of life
■ a change in bowel habits (like constipation or diarrhoea or the two alternating) or any mucus or discharge from the back passage
■ a persistent cough or hoarseness
■ any unexplained weight loss.

Point 9: Have a regular cervical smear test

■ All women who have, or have had, a sex life should have a cervical smear test (see Chapter 9). Remember that this test can detect a problem before cancer has developed and you can be completely cured.

Point 10: Examine your breasts every month

■ It really is wise, and so easy, for every woman to examine her own breasts every month. See Chapter 9 for how to do it. Remember that the vast majority of lumps are not cancer but, if cancer is present, the earlier it is discovered the greater the chance of a complete cure.

■ Take advantage, too, of mammography or X-ray examination of the breasts (see Chapter 9).

A POSTSCRIPT FOR MEN

Although it's not part of the European Code, there's something further men can do regularly and that is to examine their own testicles. Cancer of the testicles is quite rare (much less common than breast cancer in women) but it's an important cancer for two reasons: it most commonly occurs to fit young men in their prime, between the ages of 20 and 40; and it is one of the most easily cured of all cancers as today's treatments are very effective. Bob Champion, the jockey, was cured of testicular cancer and went on to ride Aldaniti to victory in the Grand National. As always, the sooner testicular cancer is detected, the greater the chance of a complete cure.

So, it is well worth getting into the habit of examining your testicles regularly – preferably every month. It will take you less than a couple of minutes.

The testicles are the male reproductive organs and they normally descend into the sac of the skin called the scrotum just before or after birth. Males whose testicles have not descended are at a slightly higher risk of developing testicular cancer so, if you find one of your testicles is missing, consult your doctor straight away.

■ Examining your own testicles is best done when the scrotal skin is relaxed, after a warm bath or shower. You need to get used to the normal feel of your testicles so that you detect any change from what is normal for you.

■ Rest your scrotum in the palms of your hands so you use the thumb and fingers of both hands to examine each testicle in turn.

■ Note the size and weight of each testicle. It's quite normal to have one testicle larger than the other (and for one to hang lower than the other) but they should both feel roughly the same weight. If one feels heavier than the other, you should consult your doctor.

- Now feel all round each testicle with your thumb and fingers. You will feel a soft tube at the top and back of each testicle. This is normal: it's called the epididymis and it stores and transports sperm. Don't confuse it with an abnormal lump.
- Check each testicle for any lumps, swellings or irregularities, any enlargement, or any change in firmness.
- If you do notice anything unusual, see your doctor as soon as possible. It is unlikely to be cancer so don't be afraid to go, but remember that if it is cancer, the chances of a cure are excellent.

11 KEEPING HEALTHY AS YOU GET OLDER

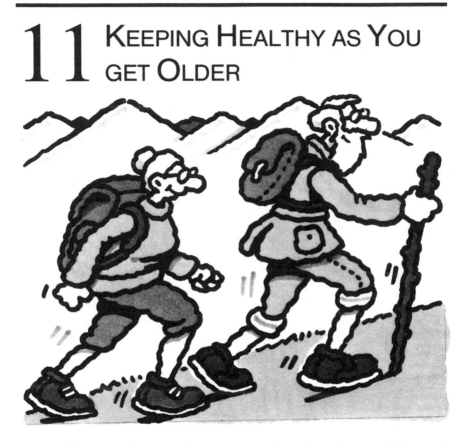

'Three score years and ten, or eighty if we have the strength' is our traditional allotted span of life. But there are now more and more people living into their eighties and nineties – and so many of them are leading full, active and healthy lives. Increasingly, people in their sixties and seventies seem no age at all. In fact, it's becoming the norm for prime ministers and presidents to be from that age group!

Age is not a disease, though some people treat it like one. Of course there are many changes that happen to you as you get older, particularly physical ones, but then, if you think about it, changes have happened to you throughout every year and decade of your life. What could be greater than the physical change from being a 10 year old to a 20 year old or, for that matter, the mental change from being a 20 year old to a 30 year old? Old age is just another stage in our life and, just as at any other stage, we can do a great deal for ourselves to help us to be healthy and lead a fuller, richer life.

To Live is to Change

Our bodies are changing every minute, every day, every year of our life. Some of the physical changes that happen as we get older are ones we'd rather do without, but there are ways of coping with them so that they cause us the least possible bother and inconvenience.

Eyesight

The lens of the eye tends to become less elastic as we get older. The eye, therefore, finds it difficult to focus and we may need glasses. But that's not unique to old age – I'm wearing them as I write this! There are two serious eye conditions which get more common as people get older: glaucoma or increased pressure in the eyeball; and cataracts, where the lens becomes more like frosted glass than clear glass. Both of these conditions can be easily and very successfully treated if caught early enough.

- Always have your eyes tested at the opticians at least once every two years.
- See your doctor immediately if you have: any pain in your eyes; if your eyesight gets bad; if you get blurred or double vision; or if you start seeing coloured haloes around lights.
- Always make sure you've got adequate lighting and strong enough light bulbs at home: if you haven't and you improve them you'll be amazed at the improvement in your eyesight!

Hearing

Most people, as they get older, find that their hearing isn't as good as it used to be. Only for a very few people does the hearing become so bad that it's a real disability. Don't accept it as normal if you're having difficulty in hearing.

■ If you're having difficulty in hearing normal conversations or the radio or television, see your doctor straight away. There may be a very simple problem – like wax in your ears – that your doctor can clear up easily.

■ Hearing aids are available free under the NHS. Think carefully and ask your doctor's advice if you want to buy a commercial one. For expert advice, contact The Royal National Institute for the Deaf or The British Association for the Hard of Hearing (addresses and phone numbers on pp. 140–1).

Hair

Virtually everyone gets grey hair as they get older and many get thinning hair or baldness as well.

■ Think of changing your hairstyle or wearing a wig. Knowing that you look good is a great morale booster.

■ If you're bald, remember that a great amount of heat is lost through the head so always wear a hat in cold weather. Be careful not to get too much sun on your scalp either (see p. 125).

Feet

Many older people are stopped from getting out and about by painful feet. Don't suffer in silence.

■ See a qualified chiropodist to get treatment which is free for pensioners on the NHS. Your doctor or nurse will make an appointment. If you go to a private chiropodist, make sure it's a state registered one.

■ Don't treat hard skin or corns yourself; ask your chiropodist who will also be pleased to cut your toe-nails if you can't do it yourself.

Teeth

About three-quarters of people in Britain have lost their teeth by the time they are in their mid-seventies. But it's not inevitable to lose our teeth as we get older.

- If you have your own teeth, brush them regularly and thoroughly using a fluoride toothpaste. See your dentist for a check-up every six months and ask for advice on keeping your teeth and gums healthy.
- If you have dentures, make sure you wear them every day as your gums can shrink if you leave them out. If they're uncomfortable see your dentist who can easily correct them so they fit properly. Have them checked every five years anyway in case they need adjusting or replacing.

IT'S YOUR AGE!

Just because there are so many physical changes with increasing age, it doesn't mean that *everything* that happens to you as you get older is because of your age. Many people do get into the way of thinking that any problem they get or any symptom they have can be put down to their age. What is worse, many doctors get into that way of thinking as well. So don't just accept the explanation 'What do you expect at your age' to any health problem that you may have.

Being overweight

It's often assumed that it's natural to put on weight as we get older: it isn't. Middle-age and old-age spread are not normal. No matter what age you are, all the advice in Chapters 1 and 2 on healthy eating and losing weight applies to you. It's true that we tend to get less active as we get older and so if we continue to eat the same amount of food, we will tend to put on weight. But again, becoming less active with age isn't an unchangeable law of the universe – we can do something about it because we are in control.

Rising blood pressure

Again it's assumed, by some doctors too, that it's natural for our blood pressure to rise as we get older: it isn't. A high blood pressure is abnormal and may be dangerous at any age. There's a great deal we can do ourselves to prevent it (see Chapter 7).

What You Can Do Yourself to Keep Healthy as You Get Older

There's so much you can do to keep yourself healthy and active right into extreme old age. Don't say 'what does it matter at my age?' It does matter. You're not trying to live forever, but you should be trying to be all you can be, no matter what age you are. Why not try to enjoy life to the full, whether you're going to live another year or another 30 years?

'You are what you eat'

This still holds true however old you are. A balanced and varied diet is essential to ensure you get all the goodness your body needs, including all the vitamins and minerals. Then you won't need anything like vitamin pills. Try to ensure you have at least one portion of the following types of food every day:

wholegrain cereals (e.g., branflakes, Weetabix, Shredded Wheat)
bread, preferably wholemeal
fresh fruit
fresh or frozen vegetables
chicken, fish, lean meat, a portion of low-fat cheese like Edam, Brie, Camembert or low-fat Cheddar
low-fat dairy products like skimmed or semi-skimmed milk or low-fat yoghurt.

And once or twice a week you can eat:

1 or 2 eggs

Go through Chapter 1 to see the changes we should all be making to turn our diet into a more healthy one:

- Eat less fat.
- Eat less sugar.
- Eat more fibre.

The first two will counter any tendency to put on weight as we get a little less active. Eating less salt is particularly important as we get older as it can contribute to high blood pressure in some people.

See p. 14 for ideas on how to liven up food using less salt. Eating more fibre is particularly important as we get older. Many old people suffer from constipation but this is helped enormously by having a good intake of fibre – it's the natural way to deal with the problem. It also helps to protect you from several bowel diseases which are more common in older people. See pp. 15–16 for ideas on how to start increasing your fibre intake today.

Always have handy some items in the store cupboard so that you can quickly have a meal or sandwich if you don't feel well enough one day to go to the shops. Some useful items are:

tuna, packed in brine not oil
sardines, packed in brine or tomato sauce
mackerel, in brine or tomato sauce
brown rice
tinned tomatoes
tins of soup
tins of fruit, packed in natural juice, not sugar or syrup.

Keep up your fluid intake. Make sure you drink regularly – water, unsweetened fruit juice, tea and coffee, skimmed milk – even if you don't feel particularly thirsty. You need two to four pints of liquid a day (about eight teacupfuls) and some older people run into problems if they don't drink enough.

The advice on sensible alcohol drinking in Chapter 5 applies too, but remember that if you're not feeling hungry, a small glass of sherry can often work wonders in giving you an appetite.

Make a pact, or a contract, with yourself if you live alone that you're always going to cook yourself at least one meal a day. Think of it as giving yourself a treat, lay the table nicely for yourself and tell yourself you deserve it.

Why not have meals two or three times a week with a friend who also lives alone. You can share the cooking and the cost, or perhaps cook one course each. It is a pleasure cooking for someone else sometimes – a pleasure you might have forgotten.

Remember that the social services department of your local council can help if you're not well or housebound. They will deliver 'meals on wheels' for you, delivering a hot meal to your door for a small charge. They'll also know of any local lunch clubs where you can make new friends as well as enjoy a good meal. Your local branch of Age Concern or Help the Aged will advise you too (addresses and phone numbers on pp. 140–1).

Exercise

Exercise is very important as you get older: 'If you don't use it, you lose it' as the maxim goes. Of course, this doesn't mean you have to play a vigorous hour of squash or run a four-minute mile! But, whatever age you are, you'll find there's some exercise that suits you and that you can fit into your life. Go through Chapter 3 on exercise and see if you can't think of some exercise you could take up. If you start thinking of excuses for not exercising you'll find some answers there too!

The most obvious exercise is walking. Try to walk somewhere every day even if it's only to the newsagents' on the corner. But then try to start a programme of regular walking, walking a little further or a little more briskly each day. Perhaps build into your walking a stretch of going uphill. Don't rush at all – always stay within comfortable limits.

Why not find out if a local leisure centre or voluntary organisation runs day or evening classes? You'll meet new friends and it's a good way of keeping fit and supple. There are often all sorts of dancing classes and there's sure to be one that suits you. Many leisure centres organise keep fit classes for older people. Ask there or at your town hall.

Think of taking up a new sport like golf or bowls. Both of these will keep you supple and improve co-ordination as well as being very enjoyable. Games like badminton and tennis can be great fun for older people as well as younger players. Don't think you're past it; just be sure to get partners who are of a similar age and standard!

What about swimming? This is a really excellent exercise for all ages and especially good for people with arthritis or aches and pains in their joints. It's never too late to learn to swim – very many people have learned in old age and you'll feel a great sense of achievement. Ask at your local baths for details of lessons for older people. There may also be special sessions where older people can swim in peace.

Smoking

It's never too late to stop smoking and it's always worth it. Remember, from Day 1 of stopping you start to reduce your risk of heart attack, stroke, bronchitis and lung cancer (see Chapter 4).

But perhaps even more importantly for older people is the effect that stopping smoking has on the *quality* of life. Giving up will help immediately with your breathing: you'll be able to do more and walk further; and you'll be far less likely to suffer from coughs and chest infections in the winter. Stopping smoking will help with the circulation in your hands and feet (nicotine restricts the blood vessels) and you won't get the pain in the legs that many older smokers get when walking. Giving up will also cut the risk of getting gangrene in the toes, which many older smokers suffer from.

Hypothermia

As we get older, it becomes easier for the temperature of our bodies to fall. Hypothermia is caused by an inability to recognise that the temperature of our surroundings is falling. Old people who can't move around very much are particularly at risk. When hypothermia sets in it doesn't mean that you actually *feel* cold but the temperature of your body starts to fall and it may go so low that you become confused, unconscious and eventually you may die. Hypothermia is, however, completely preventable if you keep your house and yourself warm.

- Close windows and doors in unused rooms and try to exclude draughts: fill in cracks in skirting and floorboards; use draught excluders and draught stoppers made of rolled-up material or sausage-shaped cushions by your doors; use heavy curtains, with thermal lining if possible, at your windows and possibly at your front door as well; cover the letterbox with a piece of thick material.
- Think of turning one of your rooms into a bed-sitting room for the winter so that you have to keep only this one room warm and cosy.
- Don't be afraid of turning on your heating. If you're worried about your bills, you'll find that the gas or electricity boards are very helpful if you talk to them in advance. You may be eligible for a heating allowance. Check at your local Social Security Office or your Citizens' Advice Bureau.

- You may be entitled to an Insulation Grant enabling you to insulate the loft and lag the hot water tank. Apply to your local council.
- Keep yourself warm by wearing several layers of thin clothing. It is warmer than one thick layer. Cover as much of your body as possible. In really cold weather, wear a hat, scarf and gloves indoors.
- Think of wearing several layers of clothing in bed. Always put on more clothes if you get up in the night. Keep a vacuum flask with a hot drink by your bedside. Use a chamberpot if you have to get up in the night. That way you don't have to walk to a cold bathroom.
- Warm the bed with an electric blanket or hot-water bottle before getting into it. Always cover hot-water bottles so you won't burn yourself.
- Remember that moving about will help the body to generate its own heat.
- Always wrap up very well with a hat, scarf, gloves and several layers of clothing when you go out in the winter.
- Make sure that you eat well; remember the body burns up food to provide it with energy and heat.

USE YOUR DOCTOR

Your doctor should always be happy to see you and to spend time discussing your problems – he gets paid more for older people, for one thing!

Discuss any problems or worries you have with your doctor. Write them down on a piece of paper so you don't forget them when you get there. Always ask if you're worried about any tablets or medicines you've been taking or if you feel you're getting side-effects from them.

In particular, always see your doctor straight away if you get any of these symptoms:

excessive thirst
unexplained weight loss
constant tiredness
giddiness or weakness
loss of appetite

loss of power in arms or legs
bleeding from any body opening
a sore or spot that won't heal
ringing in the ears
persistent pain in your lower back
abnormal breathlessness
persistent coughing
any swelling or lumps
change in bowel habits like constipation or diarrhoea or the two
    alternating
any change in bladder habits.

BE ALL YOU CAN BE

The theme of this whole book is having knowledge to take care of
your own health and putting it into action. When you're old it's
more important than ever to do this. Sometimes – kindly but
thoughtlessly – even people like health professionals start treating
old people as if they were little children again. Don't let them. Ask
questions. Show that you've got a very lively interest in your own
body and your own health. Your body is still your own and you're
responsible for it. Take care of it and it will take care of you.

USEFUL ADDRESSES

HEALTH EDUCATION
AUTHORITY,
Hamilton House,
Mabledon Place,
London WC1H 9TX
Tel. 01-631 0930

WELSH HEALTH PROMOTION
AUTHORITY,
Brunel House,
8th Floor,
2 Fitzalan Road,
Cardiff CF2 1EB
Tel. 0222-472472

SCOTTISH HEALTH
EDUCATION GROUP,
Woodburn House,
Canaan Lane,
Edinburgh EH10 4SG
Tel. 031-447 8044

DEPARTMENT OF HEALTH
AND SOCIAL SERVICES
NORTHERN IRELAND,
Dundonald House,
Upper Newtownards Road,
Belfast BT4 3SF
Tel. 0232-650111

SPORTS COUNCIL,
16 Upper Woburn Place,
London WC1H 0QP
Tel. 01-388 1277

ACTION ON SMOKING AND
HEALTH (ASH),
5–11 Mortimer Street,
London W1N 7RN
Tel. 01-637 9843

ALCOHOL CONCERN,
305 Gray's Inn Road,
London WC1X 8QF
Tel. 01-833 3471

ALCOHOLICS ANONYMOUS,
PO Box 514,
11 Redcliffe Gardens,
London SW10 9BQ
Tel. 01-352 3001

AGE CONCERN ENGLAND,
Bernard Sunley House,
60 Pitcairn Road,
Mitcham,
Surrey CR4 3LL
Tel. 01-640 5431

AGE CONCERN NORTHERN
IRELAND,
128 Great Victoria Street,
Belfast BT2 7BG
Tel. 0232-245729

AGE CONCERN SCOTLAND,
33 Castle Street,
Edinburgh EH2 3DN
Tel. 031-225 5000

AGE CONCERN WALES,
1 Park Grove,
Cardiff CF1 3BJ
Tel. 0222-371821

HELP THE AGED,
St James's Walk,
London EC1B 1BD
Tel. 01-253 0253

ROYAL NATIONAL INSTITUTE
FOR THE DEAF,
105 Gower Street,
London WC1E 6AH
Tel. 01-387 8033

BRITISH ASSOCIATION FOR
THE HARD OF HEARING,
7–11 Armstrong Road,
London W3 7JL
Tel. 01-743 1110

FURTHER READING

You might find it useful and interesting to look at the following books and leaflets:

Lynch, Dr Barry, *The BBC Diet*, BBC Books 1988

Lynch, Dr Barry, *Don't Break Your Heart*, Sidgwick & Jackson in association with BBC Wales 1987

Robertson, Ian, and Heather, Nick, *Let's Drink to Your Health!* The British Psychological Society 1986

Vessey, M. P. and Gray, Muir, *Cancer Risks and Prevention*, Oxford University Press 1987

Leaflets available from the Health Education Authority (send an s.a.e. to LAYH Pack, Department 250, 39 Standard Road, London NW10 6HD):

Guide to Healthy Eating

That's the Limit

Beating Heart Disease

Exercise, Why Bother?

A Smoker's Guide to Giving Up

General Index

adrenalin, 100
aerobic exercise, 49, 56
ageing, 130–9
alcohol, 73–88, 98, 108, 124, 135
anaerobic exercise, 49
arthritis, 18

babies
  alcohol and, 82–3
  smoking and, 61
backache, 18, 49
badminton, 57, 136
beer, 74, 75–7
bicycling, 56
  exercise bikes, 55–6
biscuits, 10, 13
blood pressure, 46, 92, 93, 94, 95–8
  see also high blood pressure
bones, osteoporosis, 46, 118, 120
bowel cancer, 15, 124–5
bread, 4
breakfast, 4, 25–6
breast cancer, 59, 113–16, 123, 124, 127–8
breathing exercises, 103–4, 105
bronchitis, 59–60
Bruce, Ken, 53
butter, 8

caffeine, 106
cakes, 10
calcium, 15, 118
cancer, 5
  alcohol and, 81
  breast, 59, 113–16, 123, 124, 127–8
  cervical, 111–12, 127
  diet and, 7, 15, 18
  lung, 59, 60, 123
  reducing risks, 121–9
  skin, 125–6
  smoking and, 59, 60
  testicles, 128–9
carbohydrates, 14

cataracts, 131,
cervical cancer, 111–12, 127
Champion, Bob, 128
cheese, 11
chemicals, cancer risks, 126–7
cholesterol, 7, 11–12, 15, 18, 46, 93, 94, 95
cigarette smoking *see* smoking
cirrhosis of the liver, 74, 81
coffee, 106
cold, hypothermia, 137–8
colon, diverticular disease, 5
COMA, 4
constipation, 5, 15, 135
contraception, 111, 117
contraceptive pills, 61, 92, 97
cream, 10
cycling, 56
  exercise bikes, 55–6

dancing, 56
deafness, 131–2
dentures, 133
diabetes, 5, 15, 18, 81, 92
diaries
  drinking diary, 76–9
  exercise diary, 43, 44
  food diary, 18–19
  smoking diary, 64–6
  stress diary, 101–2
diet
  and cancer, 124–5
  and health, 3–16, 108
  in old age, 134–6
  weight-loss, 17–28
diverticular disease, 5, 15
drinking, 73–88, 108, 124, 135
drinking water, 92
driving, drinking and, 83–4
Dunn, John, 102

eggs, 11–12
emotional problems, 100, 119

emphysema, 59–60
exercise, 43–57
    aerobic, 49, 56
    check-ups before, 47–8
    plan, 52–7
    and heart disease, 46, 48, 49, 50–1,
        93, 98
    in old age, 136
    pulse rate, 50–1
    stamina, 49
    strength, 49
    and stress, 103
    suppleness, 48
    weight loss, 23
    women, 108
exercise bikes, 55–6
eyesight, 131

fat
    cancer and, 124
    exercise and, 46
    heart disease and, 93, 98
    how to reduce, 8–12
    and old age, 134
    polyunsaturated fats, 6, 7
    saturated fats, 6–7, 93
    sources of, 7–8
    and weight loss, 17, 24, 25
feet, ageing, 132
fibre, 12, 14–16, 17, 124–5, 134–5
'fitness gap', 45
flatulence, 15
food additives, 125
food diary, 18–19
fruit, 12, 13, 15, 124–5

gallstones, 5, 15, 18
glaucoma, 131
golf, 57

hair, ageing, 132
hearing, 131–2
heart disease, 89–94
    alcohol and, 81
    diet and, 5, 7, 12, 15
    exercise and, 46, 48, 49, 50–1, 93,
        98
    mortality rates, 89–90
    overweight and, 18, 93
    risk factors, 90–4
    smoking and, 59, 60

stress and, 101
high blood pressure
    alcohol and, 81
    diet and, 5, 13
    meditation and, 105
    in old age, 133
    overweight and, 18
hormones
    hormone replacement therapy,
        119–20
    premenstrual tension, 109–10
    stress, 100, 103
hot flushes, 117–18
Hunniford, Gloria, 24
hypothermia, 137–8

impotence, 82
iron, 15

Jacobs, David, 84
Jameson, Derek, 45
jogging, 56–7

Lind, James, 3
liver, cirrhosis, 74, 81
Love, Adrian, 62
lung cancer, 59, 60, 123
lung diseases, 18, 59–60

mammography, 116, 128
margarine, 8, 25
meat, 8
meditation, 105
menopause, 60, 91, 117–20
menstruation, 109, 117
milk, 4, 9–10, 15
minerals, 15
moles, 126
monounsaturated fats, 6, 7

NACNE, 4
nervous system, alcohol and, 81
night sweats, 117–18

oestrogen, 118, 119
oils, cooking, 8–9, 25
old age, 130–9
oral contraceptives, 61, 92, 97
osteoporosis, 46, 118, 120
overweight
    cancer and, 124

diet and, 5, 7, 12
exercise and, 46–7
food diaries, 18–19
14-day weight-loss plan, 17–24
heart disease and, 18, 93
in old age, 133

pancreas, alcohol and, 81
periods, 109, 117
the 'Pill', 61, 92, 97
polyunsaturated fats, 6, 7
potatoes, 4
pregnancy, 82–3, 108
premenstrual tension, 109–11
progesterone, 119, 120
pulse rate, 50–1

relaxation, 103–5, 111
rowing machines, 55–6
Royal College of Physicians, 74
running, 56–7

salt, 13–14, 98, 134–5
saturated fats, 6–7, 93
scurvy, 3
skin cancer, 125–6
skipping, 55
slimming, 17–28
smoking, 58–72
    and cancer, 122, 123–4
    and cervical cancer, 111
    diary, 64–6
    exercise and, 46
    14-day plan for stopping, 63–72
    and heart disease, 93, 94
    and high blood pressure, 95, 98
    in old age, 137
    mortality rates, 59–60
    and oral contraceptives, 92
    women, 60–1, 92, 108
snacks, 11, 13, 19
sport, 43–57, 136
squash, 57
stamina, 49
stomach cancer, 123, 125
strength, 49

stress, 99–106, 108
    deep breathing, 103–4
    deep relaxation, 104–5
    exercise and, 46, 103
    heart disease and, 93, 98
    meditation, 105
    stress diary, 101–2
    women, 108
strokes
    alcohol and, 81
    avoiding, 95–8
    diet and, 5
    exercise and, 46
    oral contraceptives and, 92
sugar, 12–13, 17, 24
sunlight, 125
suppleness, 48
swimming, 54, 136

teeth, 132–3
tennis, 57, 136
testicles, cancer, 128–9
Thompson, Daley, 45
tranquillisers, 106

vagina, dryness, 118
vegetables, 15, 16, 124–5
vitamins, 15, 125

walking, 45, 51–2, 53, 136
weight loss, 17–28
wine, 74, 75–7
women, 107–20
    breast cancer, 59, 113–16, 123, 124,
        127–8
    cervical cancer, 111–12, 127
    drinking, 74, 78–80, 82, 108
    heart attacks, 91
    menopause, 60, 91, 117–20
    premenstrual tension, 109–11
    smoking, 60–1, 92, 108

X-rays, 116, 128

yoghurt, 10–11
Young, Jimmy, 5

INDEX OF RECIPES

almond toast, French, 29
apples
   walnut and apple salad, 38
apricot fool, 42

banana, baked, 41
beef
   chilli con carne y frijoles, 31
   pasticcio, 32
   stir-fried beef with vegetables, 30
bulgar wheat salad, 40

carrots
   carrot salad with mustard seeds, 39
   devilled carrots, 34
cashew nuts, spicy rice with, 36
chicken
   chicken pasta salad, 37
   savoury filled pancakes, 33
chilli con carne y frijoles, 31
coriander, yoghurt with walnuts and, 41
courgette, garlicky, 36

devilled carrots, 34

fish
   savoury filled pancakes, 33
French almond toast, 29
fruit salad, 41

garlicky courgette, 36
green bean salad, 38

hearty lentil soup, 29
Hollandaise sauce, 40

lentil soup, 29

macaroni
   pasticcio, 32
Mexican chilli with meat and beans, 31
mixed salad, 37

mustard seeds, carrot salad with, 39

noodles with lemon sauce, 35

okra
   prawn and okra gumbo, 34
orange and onion ring salad, 39

pancakes, savoury filled, 33
pasta, chicken salad, 37
pasticcio, 32
peas and water chestnuts, 35
prawn and okra gumbo, 34

red kidney beans
   chilli con carne y frijoles, 31
rice with cashew nuts, 36

salads
   bulgar wheat, 40
   carrot with mustard seeds, 39
   chicken pasta, 37
   green bean, 38
   mixed, 37
   orange and onion ring, 39
   salad supreme, 38
   tuna, 39
   walnut and apple, 38
sauce, Hollandaise, 40
savoury filled pancakes, 33
soup, hearty lentil, 29
spicy rice with cashew nuts, 36
stir-fried beef with vegetables, 30

tagliatelle al limone, 35
toast, French almond, 29
tuna salad, 39

walnuts
   walnut and apple salad, 38
   yoghurt with walnuts and fresh coriander, 41
water chestnuts, peas and, 35

yoghurt with walnuts and fresh coriander, 41

The following blank diaries and charts are for you to fill in following the guidelines in the book.

EXERCISE DIARY

Time	Where was I?	What did I do?

FOOD DIARY

When	Where	What	With whom

Activity	Hungry?	Mood	Comment

SMOKING DIARY   Day_____

Time	What were you doing?	Who were you with?

	How were you feeling?	How much did you enjoy it?	How much did you need it?

HOW MANY UNITS OF ALCOHOL DO YOU DRINK IN A WEEK?

Day	When	Where
	Morning Afternoon Evening	
	Morning Afternoon Evening	
	Morning Afternoon Evening	
	Morning Afternoon Evening	
	Morning Afternoon Evening	
	Morning Afternoon Evening	
	Morning Afternoon Evening	

With whom	What	Units	Total for day

Total units for week

DRINKING DIARY

Day	When	Where	With whom	What